Contents

	PROLOGUE: One busy day in the Arctic	6
1	Ireland	14
2	Vancouver Hospital and a Flying License	18
3	Flying Doc or Medical Pilot Burns Lake, Northern British Columbia	23
4	Rosie's Family	38
5	Flying to Alaska	43
6	The Arctic Beckons	50
7	Cambridge Bay, N.W.T. Living and working in the Arctic	58
8	The Inuit	66
9	Arctic Medicine, Flying, & a Snowmobile Trip	90
10	Unusual Medical Problems in the North	97
11	Infanticide: immoral or necessity?	104
12	Medevacs and Arctic Flying	108
13	Isolation	117
14	Explorers, Anthropologists and Priests	124
15	Cambridge Bay to Cambridge University	132
16	Nanisivik, Baffin Island	137
17	Return to the Arctic	140
18	Tuktoyaktuk	146
	EPILOGUE	158

Acknowledgements

Writing a book has some similarity to flying. Both are adventures; both have their good times and their challenges; perhaps most important, both have their unsung heroes. In flying, ground crews, navigators, weather experts, radio operators and the support and skill of the co-pilot come to mind. In writing, in order for the mission to be successful, similar systems of support are necessary.

This book was drafted in rough form in 1983. It was not until the particularly snowy winter of 1996, following my move to Nelson B.C., that I was able to finish it. It proved to be an exciting challenge, and I want to express my thanks to an amazing "ground crew"! Elizabeth Fleet offered extensive advice as editor and proof reader. Anne De Grace put me in touch with Fiona Richardson and Doug Jones, talented graphic designers; and Angela Lockerbie, who helped with camera-ready peparation. My friend and fellow pilot, David Gluns, helped me with photos. Pat MacIntosh, Mae Hooper, and Brenda Lee read the manuscript and gave moral support. Final decisions in the preparation of the book were my own, and I remain responsible for any errors.

It has been an exciting, busy and challenging journey. Most of all my thanks and appreciation are expressed to my wife and "co-pilot" in this adventure, Diana Haschke, who has always been fully supportive.

Foreword

Doctors and pilots enjoy making decisions and the Canadian North provides many situations requiring unusual solutions. I took my medical training in Ireland and worked both there and in England before heading off to Vancouver in 1970. Shortly thereafter, I tried my hand at a "Flying Doctor" job in Burns Lake, a small community in northern British Columbia. It was the Arctic, however, which presented the most formidable challenges, and my experiences there form the focus for most of this book.

The terms "Eskimo" and "Inuit" are used without prejudice. The correct word, in the context of this book, was "Eskimo". This word comes from an Algonquian Indian word meaning "eater of raw meat." It was the accepted word in English, for the northern peoples, until the Eskimo language word "Inuit" came into more accepted usage.

The word "Inuit" means "The People." In Inuktitut, the language of the Inuit, "whites" are referred to as "Kabloonaks," meaning "those with bushy eyebrows." In this book the term "white" is used to refer to all non-Inuit people, as was the custom of the time. Place names have changed since the seventies, but the commonly used names of the times appear in this book.

Many of us go north to find ourselves; to challenge ourselves, to seek adventure, or to escape the humdrum of southern life. While pursuing my career, I too was seeking answers; searching in a way not always possible in our normal lives. It is my hope that in recapturing the memories of this time there is something of a story to be told, for others to enjoy.

Prologue

ONE BUSY DAY IN THE ARCTIC

SUNDAY AUGUST 21ST 1974: 6 P.M.
DIARY ENTRY:
CAMBRIDGE BAY.

Just finished four tiring days when I get a call from Sue Dobson, one of two nurses in Gjoa Haven, over three hundred miles away from Cambridge Bay where I am based. I am at this time the most northerly physician in Canada; a dubious claim to fame. My nearest source of professional help, excluding nurses, is Yellowknife Hospital, five hundred and forty miles south. Telephones have only recently been installed in Gjoa Haven.

"Dr. Dale, I need a plane over here. I have a lady with acute abdominal pain; spasmodic. She seems to be in shock but has a normal blood pressure. She has generalized abdominal tenderness and pain. There are no localizing signs."

It sounds like a surgical abdomen, although we cannot be sure of a diagnosis yet. Sue does not panic easily and if she requests a plane I do not question it.

"O.K. Sue, I'll get a plane as soon as I can, but there is nothing available here. It will mean getting one up from Yellowknife to collect me enroute."

Sue will start an IV and give the patient some morphine if needed, as we have many hours to wait. Now I have to make the decision as to which plane to use. In a dire emergency I could divert a passenger jet, but generally we are able to locate a Twin Otter. "Medevacs" are still in their infancy, as far as equipment, so I use my own pre-packed emergency medical bag.

If I call for a plane, nobody questions my decision, just

as I do not argue with nurses out in the distant communities. We are on the spot, guessing at diagnoses with very few of the amenities of modern medicine. We can do a complete white cell count and test urine and we do have X-ray machines. That is about it however, and we have to rely heavily on clinical intuition.

The Arctic can be a cold, distant, lonely place, but never so much as when it takes eighteen hours to evacuate an acutely ill patient. Sue will try to keep the patient comfortable, but it is frustrating to cope with the long waiting period. We are at the mercy of weather and planes.

It forces me to realize how spoilt we were down south. In those days, if the haemoglobin dropped a little, we would get some blood; we don't even have blood available up here. We give Ringer's Lactate and oxygen, and hope for the best on long flights at sub-zero temperatures. IV's can freeze in between leaving the Nursing Station and arriving at the airport. The "ambulance" might be an actual pickup, with the patient bundled in sleeping bags, or a sled behind a skidoo, or, if we are lucky, we travel in a Nodwell. The Nodwell is an enclosed snow machine, capable of carrying eight passengers. It runs on tracks and has the suspension of a tank! Sometimes the "road" is almost impassable and then a very bumpy ride ensues. There is often no question of being able to hang an IV bottle. It has to go inside our jackets, as does most of the IV line. They both tended to freeze quickly. I wonder if someone could die from a fast moving ice embolus!

Many physicians find this aspect of the job too frustrating; I find it humbling. To me it is amazing what the human body will endure, and sometimes recover from, without all the technological aid on which we depend so much.

The Twin Otter arrives at Cambridge Bay at 3 a.m. After gassing up we head over to Gjoa Haven.

Enroute, the throb of the PT-6 engines lulls me into a reverie. I gaze at the flat, flat ground beneath me, now free of snow. Ahead is the sea ice between Victoria Island and King William Island; I shiver looking at it. It is mid-summer but I feel cold just looking at this frigid landscape. I am trying to define the appeal; the magic of this Arctic experience. The seats on a Twin Otter are not very comfortable but I am drifting in and out of slumber. Yet, in between episodes of sleep, I am as aware as ever of the excitement I feel at being up in this part of the world. I gaze out of the left window of the plane. Somewhere within eyesight, Franklin's ships were abandoned, just 127 years ago. At the turn of the century, Amundsen sailed through this very passage which is passing beneath my right wing, often fighting his way through ice floes. There seems to be an instant contact through the ages to past history. If, at those times, they had been able to look down from 10,000 feet, the scenery would have been identical. That surely is part of the magic.

Nervousness about this particular patient forces me back to the present. It is evident that we are dealing with a surgical emergency. This is fine, but we are many hours from a hospital. My total surgical skills amount to a bunch of orthopaedic operations on legs and hips, one or two appendix operations and one C-Section. I am not able to perform this kind of surgery. I am probably totally unqualified for this job! I expect everyone, in this job, has these doubts.

A call to the surgeon in Yellowknife confirms my suspicion that we are dealing with an intestinal obstruction. We depart for Yellowknife. Enroute, due to my ignorance of the effect of altitude on medical emergencies, the poor woman gets into incredible pain before I remember that air trapped in an obstruction will expand. Stupid! I ask the pilot to stay at 2000 feet above ground; the patient settles somewhat. However, now she does become shocked and I am only able to assist with IV fluids. We do not land until 5 p.m. She is operated on later and has a volvulus; a form of twisted bowel. She does just fine.

I have flown over one thousand miles and been up since 1 a.m. I sleep well in a hotel that night; travelling back next morning to Cambridge Bay—on top of flour sacks—in the back of a cargo Twin Otter.

The return flight takes four hours and as soon as I am home, and say 'hi' to my wife, I am off again on a Twin Otter on floats, to do the summer check down at Bay Chimo. The Inuit are out at their summer camps. The Bathurst Inlet area is one of the most beautiful settings in the world; it is no wonder the local Inuit seem happier than many others.

There are perhaps fifty permanent Inuit in this area. In summer, a camp run by an ex-RCMP and his wife provides employment for quite a few families. During that glorious but short season, the remaining Inuit move out to various summer camps around the bay. They catch fish by the thousands and dry them on clothes lines for three or four days. There are no flies to bother the process. The men hunt seals, the women look after the camp and the children, and the long, warm days are enjoyed by all. This is the happiest time of the year.

We fly to Fowler Bay and Brown Sound, then on to Perry Bay and Bathurst Inlct itself. After that we make a quick visit to Arctic Sound and finally to Hope Bay. I've put in eighteen hours in a plane in three days but still manage to get some right-seat time in the Twin Otter. In between I get some sleep in the back.

This area abounds with history. The place names reflect the early explorers, or their sponsors, or some adventure: Coronation Gulf, Turnagain Point, Starvation Bay, Ross Strait, Terror Bay. Just north of here is the final part of the Northwest Passage, which remained unconquered until Amundsen went through it in 1903-05. Sir John Franklin made several journeys in this area, originally by canoe. He finally died not far north of this spot.

The Inuit love it here in the Bay Chimo area; the hunting is superb and the scenery consists of rolling hills, splashed with colour. In summer, temperatures rise to pleasantly warm; the children can swim in the rivers. I am taken out to see the "Hikhik" or ground squirrels. They pop out of the ground everywhere. The whole world comes alive here in summer—it is such a contrast to the barren, cold, dark winters.

The Inuit here are self confident and almost have the best of both worlds. In close touch with all the traditional ways of hunting, they can also go to work on oil rigs. The parents seem to accept openly that their children should go to Cambridge Bay or Yellowknife for their schooling. I became good friends with the Hakungak family; George, who is just a teenager, and his Mom, May. The two of them moved up to Cambridge Bay, partly because George can go to school there and partly because May gets better poker games.

I do my various medical checks, but this is not work—it is a complete life style. I do not know what brought me up here, but I am humbled before this vast inspiring lunar landscape and its confident, happy inhabitants. Many times I wonder why I left a more predictable doctor's practice in the south. Medicine here involves social anthropology and is not just fixing a given ailment. It is a unique challenge, which ends up being the most intense period of my life. My own personal attachment to the Arctic was to go on for the next five years, and I still managed to return for some flying trips, with my own plane, in later years.

The trail which lead eventually to the Far North had its origins in Ireland in the late 1960's.

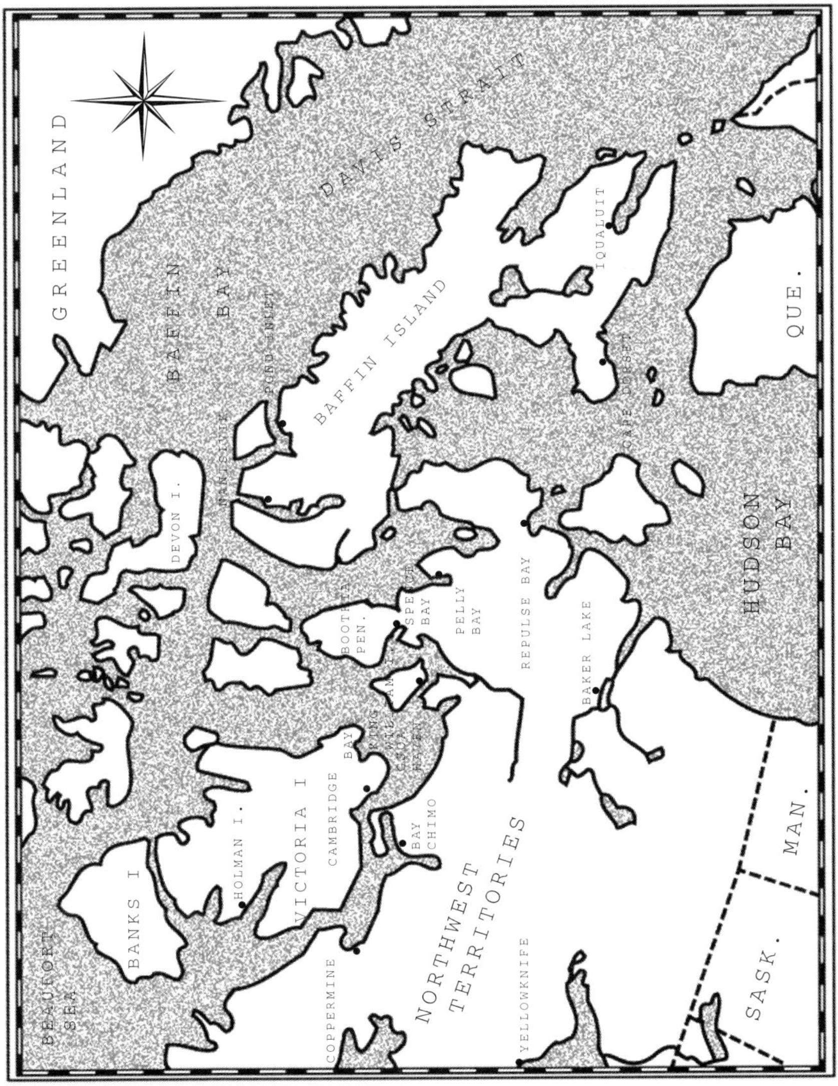
GREENLAND
BAFFIN BAY
DAVIS STRAIT
BAFFIN ISLAND
POND INLET
IQUALUIT
CAPE DORSET
QUE.
DEVON I.
HUDSON BAY
REPULSE BAY
BAKER LAKE
PELLY BAY
SPENCE BAY
BOOTHIA PEN.
CAMBRIDGE BAY
VICTORIA I
HOLMAN I.
BAY CHIMO
BANKS I
BEAUFORT SEA
COPPERMINE
NORTHWEST TERRITORIES
YELLOWKNIFE
MAN.
SASK.

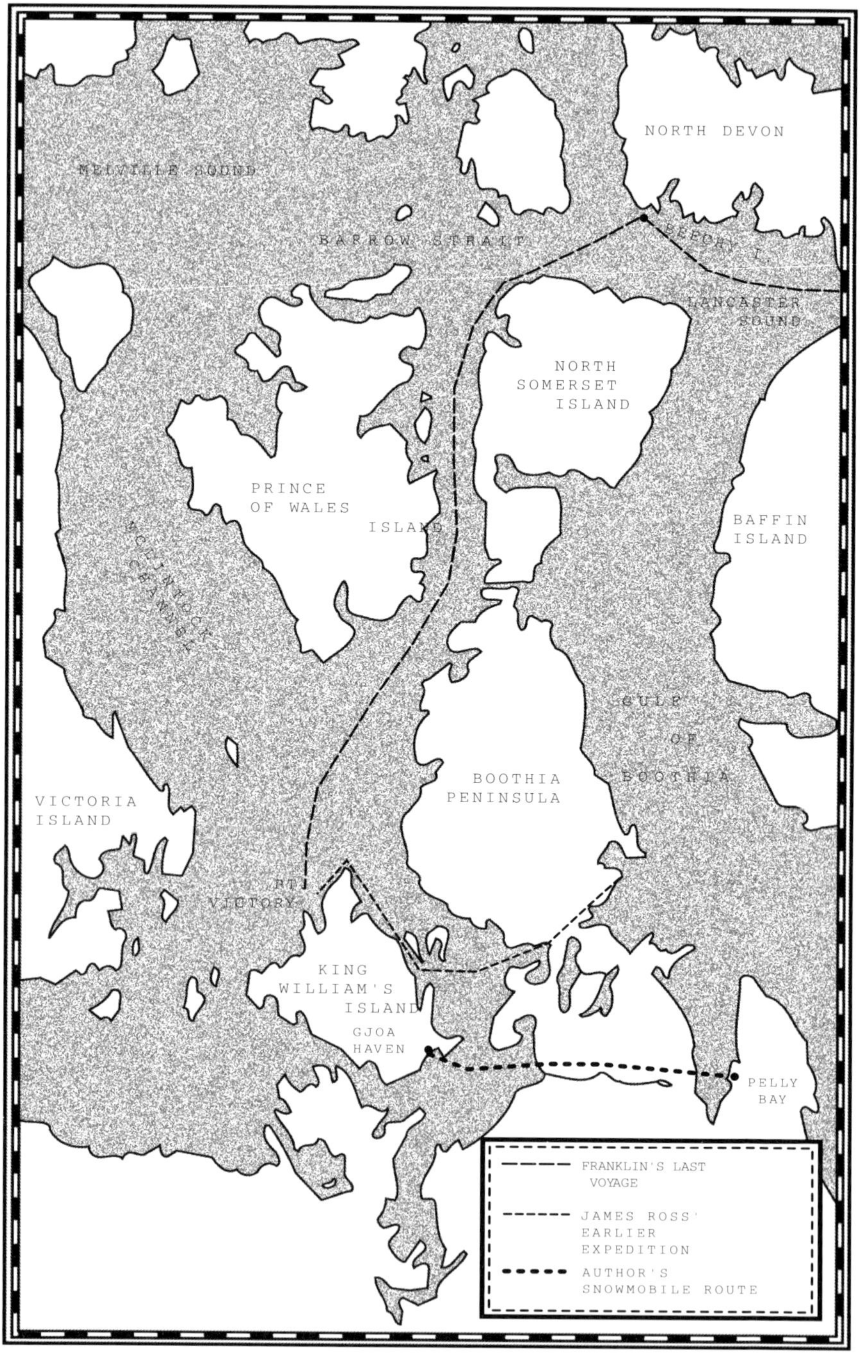
NORTH DEVON
MELVILLE SOUND
BARROW STRAIT
BEECHY I.
LANCASTER SOUND
NORTH SOMERSET ISLAND
PRINCE OF WALES ISLAND
BAFFIN ISLAND
M'CLINTOCK CHANNEL
GULF OF BOOTHIA
BOOTHIA PENINSULA
VICTORIA ISLAND
PT. VICTORY
KING WILLIAM'S ISLAND
GJOA HAVEN
PELLY BAY
FRANKLIN'S LAST VOYAGE
JAMES ROSS' EARLIER EXPEDITION
AUTHOR'S SNOWMOBILE ROUTE

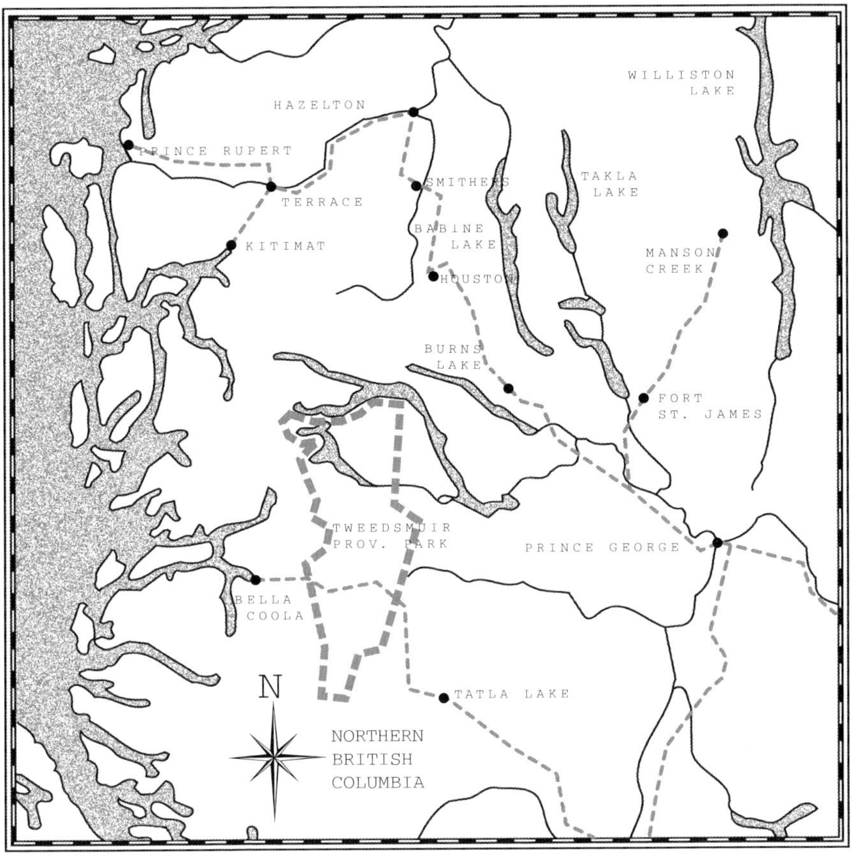

WILLISTON
LAKE
HAZELTON
PRINCE RUPERT
SMITHERS
TAKLA
LAKE
TERRACE
BABINE
LAKE
KITIMAT
MANSON
CREEK
HOUSTON
BURNS
LAKE
FORT
ST. JAMES
TWEEDSMUIR
PROV. PARK
PRINCE GEORGE
BELLA
COOLA
N
TATLA LAKE
NORTHERN
BRITISH
COLUMBIA

Chapter 1

IRELAND

Summer of 1968 - Belfast.

C-r-r-rack!............... a short burst of sub-machine fire went zinging, right above my head, into the brick walls of the Royal Victoria Hospital in Belfast.

All through the day we could see signs that there would be some excitement. Shops were boarded up; a feeling of tension was evident. The hospital was between Grosvenor Road and Falls Road, slap bang in the middle of the subsequent war zone. As yet there had been no overt violence, so we did not know how bad it was to become. I was in my final year of medical school at the Royal College of Surgeons in Ireland, located in Dublin and had come to visit a friend; a doctor at the Royal Victoria Hospital.

During the day we had wandered along the Grosvenor Road and shopkeepers just told us that they expected some minor rioting that night. When I had stepped outside the hospital for a look at things that evening, I was not expecting to be shot at. I thought initially that this was nearby firecrackers, but bits of brick came down on my head, and I soon realized that this was caused by bullets, probably from a Thompson sub-machine gun. I disappeared back inside the safety of the hospital as fast as I could.

Following the declaration of "Free Belfast" by the IRA, we stayed inside the hospital for a few days. During daytime it was safe to wander around a little. As I could not work in the hospital, I had some spare time and was able to talk to participants on either side of the barricades. Across Grosvenor Road were burnt out buses, still smouldering, being used as barricades. Private militia guarded the entrance, but by disguising my English accent I gained entrance through the barricades.

"Who started all this fighting?" I asked innocently.

"Those Protestant bastards!" came the reply.

They were referring primarily to the B-Specials, a branch of the Royal Ulster Constabulary. They were not well liked by the Catholics.

Horror stories of unprovoked shooting were related with passionate language. I peered across the barricades to the far side of the street, to make sure that no unprovoked shooting took place while I was there. It seemed fair to go and hear the other version. Prudence dictated that I walk a few hundred yards down the road first. There were overturned buses, and some burnt out bread vans. Every single street was blocked off and barricaded. This time I assumed a more English accent:

"Who started all this?" I asked, pointing to bullet holes, upturned vehicles and even a blood stain on the wall.

"Those IRA bastards!"

This was then followed by further stories of unjustified terror and violence. I returned to the hospital glad that I was not personally involved in this weird, religious and political strife, but realizing that it would not go away for a long time. In 1922, when Lloyd George divided the country into Ulster and Eire, he created a compromise solution. Now we were in a conflict, partly religious, partly economic, fuelled by international terrorism and lunatics.

I returned to my studies in Dublin and finished my medical degree. My interest in philosophy was developing more and more. After graduation, I tried for a loan from the bank to continue my studies into Immanuel Kant. Whilst a student I had been fortunate to meet Dr. Con Drury. He had been a student of Ludwig Wittgenstein, in the early thirties, at Cambridge University. My own studies had included two years of Bertrand Russell and some Wittgenstein. My introduction to Dr. Drury had come about in an unusual manner. In one exam in physiology I was being examined by Professor Kane. Initially he asked me a few physiology questions then peered at a book which I was carrying and said:

"Is that a Bertrand Russell book I see?"

"Yes Sir," said I, feeling happy that I had at least one answer right. Then I started to feel nervous, thinking that he might perceive my lack of interest in medical studies as a serious problem. My nervousness increased as I remembered that Prof. Kane was a cunning old devil. He was probably asking a deep existential question and I had given a superficial answer. Had I failed to comprehend his comment on the nature of reality? Would I now be given an erudite exposition on the epistemological ramifications of my glib answer? Luckily this all proved to be neurotic thinking!

"Excellent," he said. "I read 'Principia Mathematica,' or parts thereof."

We followed up with a discussion on Wittgenstein after which Prof. Kane gave me an introduction to Con Drury who, at that time, was running a small mental hospital at Lucan, just outside Dublin.

I passed the physiology exam with no more questions on physiology! The introduction to Drury gave me many years of pleasant discussion and useful further contacts in philosophy.

After my own graduation, finances dictated that I find a job. I felt ill-prepared for working as a doctor, and would rather have gone on with philosophy; however, if I had to work it might as well be somewhere new and interesting, so I chose Northern Ireland, or Ulster, rather than England. I applied to a small hospital in Coleraine, not too far from Londonderry.

The British troops were in Ulster now, but Coleraine was in a fairly peaceful area; meanwhile the battle continued in Belfast. On one occasion I had to escort a patient with a sub-arachnoid haemorrhage and stayed overnight at the Royal Victoria with my friend, Jessin, who was now a qualified obstetrician. We watched the nightly show of burning buildings from an upper floor in the hospital. Machine guns popped off at intervals; five dead that night and one hundred injured. Shotguns and petrol bombs were used and on occasions young doctors were "borrowed" from the hospital and returned later by the IRA.

The six months in Coleraine passed quickly, helped by lots of on-call and occasional visits to the local pub! I received a call from a friend about a possible job at the Royal Sussex County Hospital in Brighton. There was a need for a house-surgeon in Accident and Orthopaedic Surgery. It seemed like a good idea to try working in England, though I was apprehensive about fitting in after my time in Eire and Ulster. Brighton offered a good social life and an enjoyable learning experience in Emergency Medicine. I was able to start my flying license at nearby Shoreham. In the meantime I decided that I would go to British Columbia after this job ended, and applied for a residency in paediatrics at the Children's Hospital in Vancouver. I knew that flying was cheaper in Canada!

Chapter 2

VANCOUVER HOSPITAL AND A FLYING LICENSE

On arrival in Vancouver, in June of 1970, I was thrown into the deep end of a busy residency training in paediatrics. To escape from the hospital was hard; to switch off and relax, even harder. My soul was desolate here with this first introduction to Canada. After six months I had made the decision to quit the program. Perhaps I was not strong enough emotionally to go through the trauma of coping with little children dying. Many had leukaemia and helping to look after them drained me. Maybe it was easier for other doctors to work in this area; I found it very hard. The balance between satisfying a desire to help those who suffer and the amount one is able to give to that ambition is a difficult one for doctors.

Selfishly, I wanted more from life than medicine alone; I wanted to fly and read more philosophy. Then there was research. Whilst I could agree it had to happen, I did not like to cause little children the pain necessary to continue research. The parents were stronger than I was, knowing that their children were using an experimental drug, or receiving intra-thecal injections, i.e. into the spinal canal, every week. I still had to perform the procedure, knowing the children would die anyway.

In the future, other children might benefit from this research. I tried to hide my trepidation as I walked down the corridor to give yet another spinal injection into some little child. Even with sedation the little mites would know what was coming.

One lovely, courageous six year old girl had advanced cystic fibrosis. I felt that I would happily switch places with her. I had already lived twenty-six years and here she was on her way out at six. We did not feel that it was fair to her or to her parents to resuscitate her one more time with her severe lung problems. Each infection would tire her more and more. Finally, after much discussion among relatives and doctors, we felt that the most humane decision was not to treat her next pneumonia. Yet, with her parents, we still had to watch her die.

In the next ward was Mona, aged two, with severe hydrocephalus. Minor degrees were correctable even then, by channelling the excess cerebro-spinal fluid into a vein. For Mona we could do no more. She loved music and someone had given her a little transistor radio by her pillow. If it was turned off she would get grumpy and cry. She would not go to sleep without the radio on. She died that fall. It seemed like a relief, but a little of every doctor and nurse died with her.

In Vancouver General, we would be in by 6.30 a.m., do rounds on the patients until 8.30 a.m. and then do new admissions. After that; case presentations, lunch (very brief) and continue through until 5 p.m. This was on days off. On call days we could expect to work through until midnight or 2 a.m.; an eighteen hour day was not unusual. In the first few months there, several of us complained that we did not feel we could learn much with every second night on call. This was a revolutionary concept; that it might actually be hard to remain a human being with so little sleep. There was much opposition, both from older doctors who had been through the mill and from some younger ones who felt they might miss an important case by not being there!

A DAY OFF: *Looking from the Simon Fraser Memorial out over the North Arm Jetty across the Fraser river on a Saturday afternoon. Sense of peaceful solitude. People draw up in their cars and campers—then stop for a few moments to take in the water and logs and mountains—then restless, move on. I sit and listen to the sound of the tug-boats, permeating up from the water, over a lazy summer afternoon. Bees buzz in the shrubs and I see ducks out on the water. After a while nature's peace, beauty and strength calm me back down from the pressures of the work. I sense the timelessness and imagine the Indians here, back over the centuries.*

Back at work I escape from the ward to the animal research lab, whenever I can. Firstly I finish my rounds up in "Children's Ward," then down to assist on a Fascia Lata graft to the thoracic aorta of a dog. The dogs are, of course, anaesthetized and I can handle even their sorrowful whimpering after watching what we go through with the children upstairs. The first dog has problems with the intra-luminal shunt but is recovering O.K. from the gas of the anaesthetic. The second puppy dies from a ruptured aorta and pulmonary oedema (fluid on lungs).

Nearby here is a little old lady who buys up as many dogs as she can, to prevent us from getting them from the pound. I feel that she should come in and watch some children die. We try to be as humane as possible with the animals but have, of course, made the arrogant assumption that we are more important then they are.

<u>SEPT. 20TH, 1970</u>: *Flying again, I'm in heaven out at Pitt Meadows airport, flying an old Fleet Canuck. It may be hard to learn flying but it seems like pure relaxation to me after work. Walter Borodola, my instructor, seems more worried than I am, as we wander from side to side across the runway on landings and take-offs.*

<u>SEPT. 24TH</u>: *Cardiac Surgery: My sister, Janet, and I are in the operating room together. She moved to Vancouver several years before me, and has been working as an OR nurse. Dr. Phil Ashmore and Dr. Graham Fraser are performing the surgery. I am a junior assistant here and my sister gives me a bad time, but I am too nervous to enjoy the humour. We have two long cases, the first a tetralogy of Fallot, with multiple congenital anomalies. The second is a case of total anomalous venous drainage. These are both*

congenital conditions and serious ones and sadly they both die afterwards. My admiration for the skills of all the staff is high, but I do not think this kind of work is for me.

NOV. 10TH: *Have decided to quit the training. Not quite sure why; tied up with maintaining intellectual ability to think, my personal sensitivity and creativity. Definitely a sense of failure. I tell them that I am quitting for personal reasons—they ask no more. I have to stay until New Year.*

TODAY'S ITINERARY: *Ward rounds 7.45 a.m. repeat at 8.15 with staffmen (senior doctors), twenty-five children in right now. Ten have leukaemia. Busy till lunch; quick sandwich; admit patients until 5.30... quick pizza. Four more admissions after: Noonan's syndrome (rare chromosomal abnormality), chronic recurrent urethritis, acute leukaemia, with the poor little mite vomiting blood, then a little boy with some object stuck deep into his hand.*

In between... trying to read up for a presentation, to be given the next day, on a new drug for asthma. Busy until 2 a.m., then sleep until 7.30 a.m. Thank God! Start rounds again and so forth until 3 p.m., a lucky early finish today. There is no life in between work like this. My humanity is stifled; I feel lonely. I cannot even study philosophy as it requires some peace of mind.

I thought about returning to Britain but I did not like giving up altogether and I hadn't even finished my flying license.

There was an ad on the notice board in our residence. It said: "Doctor wanted in Burns Lake. General practice. Interest in planes a help." Worth a call anyway! I hadn't been farther than Whistler yet.

"Hi! I'd like to come up and see the place and consider working for you. I don't have much experience."

" Do you have a plane?"

"No, but I'm getting my license."

"O.K. We have a runway a few miles out of town and you can finish up your license after you move here."

With that, our detailed interview was over. I was not sure if Dr. Doug Mann had any idea if I was suitable as a doctor, but for sure he knew I liked planes! It seemed a good idea to travel up and take a look at this place.

Chapter 3

FLYING DOC OR MEDICAL PILOT?

NOV. 1970: *Jet to Prince George. All of a sudden I see an incredible country unfolding beneath me. I had no idea that all this empty space was here! Sure I'd looked on maps but I had no idea of this vast, seemingly uninhabited sparseness. I am overtaken by a feeling of tremendous excitement, as I gaze at this landscape which is now covered in a blanket of white snow. Small towns pass by, then more trees; snow; trees; snow. Land at Prince George and there to meet me is a rather disreputable character in jeans, who ambles over to me:*

"You Dr. Dale?"

"Yes."

I made the assumption that he had sent a driver. This was impressive, but he could have had him dress a little better!

"Hi, I'm Doug, how do you do?"

When I realised this was the doctor I relaxed and thought that this would be a great place for me because I was such a misfit anyway. It was the first time that I had seen a doctor wearing jeans! His car was an old Ford Rambler station wagon, which had definitely seen better days. We drove the 140 miles to Burns Lake, mostly discussing flying, and I gleaned something about the job. The College of Physicians had called me in to discuss the peculiar situation in Burns Lake, as it seemed the two doctors there did not get along together.

We arrived at Burns Lake following a drive which, many years later, still manages to excite me as much as on that first journey north. Next, we took a look around town. Generally the first impression of these northern towns is one of a few gas stations and dirty streets. I was filled with a mystical wonder at this winter scene. After cities, this looked like heaven. It was like the quintessential Christmas card scene. We crossed the tracks towards the old part of town; deep snow covering everything but the twin tracks of the railway, making the driving quiet. The only sound to be heard was the noise of the tires, making that characteristic crunching sound, known only to those who have experienced the cold, dry winters of the north. We drove on down to the lake. I already felt that here a person would be recognized as an individual and my soul began to feel at peace after the turmoil of Vancouver.

There was no question in my mind about taking the job, but to make sure, Doug took me out to see his plane. It was an old Super Cub, awaiting its winter skis. The plane badly needed a coat of paint and was sitting, beached, at the edge of the lake after the float season. The letters on the plane were CF-NSF, fairly indicative of the financial implications of flying! We went on out to the airport, thirteen miles west. At this time the runway was grass and 4000' long; deserted but for Don Payne's Super Cub on wheels. This runway looked big enough for me to make all kinds of mistakes. I would need lots of space!

Next we visited the hospital, which had thirty-five beds. It was a small, friendly hospital and I felt immediately welcomed. In those days any doctor willing to move north was welcome. I would be the third doctor in town and that would mean a one in three call, which seemed heaven after one in two.

The following six weeks in Vancouver passed very slowly. In the New Year as I drove north, I felt I was emerging from a cocoon of the past. Somewhere around the beginning of the Fraser Canyon, as the haze of the lower mainland began to fade, my coastal mood and personality disappeared. I felt infinitely free of concerns and could breathe more easily.

I started work in Burns Lake in January of 1971. For the first while I was busy and heavily involved with a broad range of medical problems.

JAN. 1971: *A list of occurrences over the past few days. Day 1 on call: Rounds, at a respectable 9 a.m.! Then to the clinic, then drive up to the hospital to watch a delivery; it has been a while for me. Odd calls in the night, nothing too stressful, almost pleasantly relaxed night call after Vancouver. Next day assisting cholecystectomy for three hours. Doug does it and I am impressed at the multiple talents of these northern doctors.*

My training would have been so different if I knew I would end up here. Dr. George Magee does the anaesthetic; Dr. Doug Mann the surgery on this case but they barely talk to each other. It seems the College was right. There is a real personality difference, I resolve to try and stay neutral if possible. From then on it is decided that I should do the anaesthetics. I have never done any!!

After the surgery, I rush off to treat a young girl with an acute asthmatic attack and then have to do a delivery. It is an Indian lady and she is so relaxed she does it all for me. Says nothing; no complaint of pain, a little push and there is a baby. I think if they can all be like this, I might avoid all those horror stories from my training. Some hope!

Back to the O.R. This time I have to give an anaesthetic as George is busy elsewhere. Well I may as well learn now as ever. I have not intubated before, so the first attempt goes into the stomach. Doug has to unglove and bail me out. After that I just follow instructions.

On Friday we do rounds, read all our own X-rays, then I have a circumcision to do, then to the clinic. An Indian lady wants pills to "have more babies". An examination reveals probable V.D. and I have the lab test done in our own clinic lab, then treat her with penicillin IM. She almost killed her last baby, apparently, by trying to cure an umbilical hernia with a knitting needle. In the end I give her some birth control pills and more penicillin. After that she seems happy.

The winter here was different from any winters I had ever known. The snow fell and fell. I had never seen so much; it was beautiful. I lived up above the main highway in a rental house belonging to Doug. In the night it was so quiet, I would hear only the whistle of the freight train.

FEB. 1971: *The sun comes up over the white lake illuminating five inches of fresh snow perched on the balcony. There is a mist or ice fog over the distant valley. Every day reveals a new image and I never tire of watching. This must be what Thoreau felt in the excitement and naiveté of Walden.*

Chief "T," a local chief from Babine Lake (such wonderful names; I cannot wait to go and see all these places), has one leg, boozes like hell and gets paid every time he needs a trip to the doctor. This happens frequently as we are situated right next to the liquor store. He gets $100 each month for being chief and explains to me that he is a "Red Panther". This was in the era of the "Black Panther" movement in the States, so he is up with the times.

I started flying again as soon as I could, at Smithers with Walt Weslowski, who instructed in Langley in the summer and relaxed up in Smithers in the winter. We used a Cherokee 140 and, on my first solo, I got "lost" and happened to be buzzing over Burns Lake, right down on the ice, at four feet above it. Some friends were ice-fishing there. What a sense of freedom! Upon my arrival back at Smithers, Walt asked how my first cross country went and I said:

"Fine, though I was a little off course." He just smiled; he knew perfectly well where I had been!

Of course I had to buy a snowmobile. I purchased a Skiroule 500, wide track. Now I could explore the area around Burns Lake, where there were so many trails. One day, heading north, I ran into a crazy old hermit named Frank. He lived in a lean-to made of tarpaulin, enduring temperatures down to -50° Fahrenheit. Frank was a schizophrenic version of Ralph Nader; he lived off the garbage dump all winter. In summer he apparently hitch-hiked around, cleaning up garbage from the roads. He would get mad if people burned their garbage before he got a chance to check it out. Moose would come directly to his tent and feed with him. I watched from afar one day and could not believe anyone could survive that long out in the cold. He would light a fire of scrap wood in the tarpaulin tent for some warmth.

The RCMP deported poor old Frank after he pulled a knife on a friend of mine, who was throwing stuff away and starting to burn it. This would have only served to confirm his theory, which he explained to me one day when I gave him a lift on the snowmobile, that there was a plot against him. Trudeau had frozen Frank's brain in order to brainwash him. Now Trudeau and the RCMP were infiltrating heroin spores into the atmosphere, and these were floating down into people's brains. He was immune because he was strong.

"How do you keep up with world affairs Frank?"

"It all just comes to me," he said with certainty.

I asked him once what he thought of doctors and got a quick angry response, so I never did tell him what I did for a living. I often gave him rides on my machine and, after he was deported, I felt really sad at the thought of him locked in some mental institution, taking anti-psychotics and loosing the freedom of this beautiful harsh life. Out here at Keager Lake, the moose came right to him and he always struck me as a gentle crazy man. Getting upset with someone burning HIS garbage was quite logical.

By February I was dreaming of my flying license and had already picked my first plane. This was a Champion Citabria. For me the plane had to be aerobatic, capable of going on skis, have a good engine and good short field performance. Super Cubs are excellent but not aerobatic; they were, however, considered to be the superior bush planes. The Citabria cruised at around 125 mph and was actually more roomy than the Cub. I had to finish my license first but decided to go ahead and order the plane.

I had to drive 180 miles for each flying lesson, but it

was a gorgeous drive, through Houston and Telkwa to Smithers, and it put me in the mood to enjoy flying over the mountains. Once up in the Cherokee it was a different world. At times there was a halo in the front of the plane, from the propeller. Through this one would see white-tipped mountains and glaciers; a world of magic.

APRIL 1971: *In April I do my dual and solo cross country flight, most of my training with Walt Weslowski. Some days, after my long drive, the weather closes in and Walt calls it a Whisky Front and pulls out scotch or rye from under the chesterfield. I have to go and eat a big meal to be safe for the drive home! When the weather is good, the route for cross country flying is beautiful. Students go from Smithers through the Telkwa Pass to Terrace. There we have cheeseburgers and fly back via the Yellowhead Highway. The air is smooth, no clouds, and at 5000' the surrounding mountains dwarf us. Mt. Brian Boru at 8250' makes you squint into the sun to see the peak. Below us is a sheet of perfect white; trees showing crisply through. The trip is over much too quickly!*

All these place names up here are filled with the magic of history. Reading Father Morice's book "The History of the Northern Interior of British Columbia," brings everything alive for me. The local Carrier Indians can be seen with new respect and some understanding gained of the position modern trading, commercialism and religion, have left them. They share with the Inuit, as I learn later, an ability to survive many hardships in the environment, but a marked fatalism in their contact with a technologically superior culture. There is a certain lack of adaptability to modern social life. It is not surprising, when one considers that the Indian's primary survival skills have been adapting, over thousands of years, to environmental climate changes.

Father Morice, (1859-1938) was a man of many talents; linguist, anthropologist, historian. He was an Oblate missionary and was sent up to Fort St. James in 1885. There he gave the Athapascan people a written language. He designed one for the Carriers of Stuart Lake as well, to allow them to read bibles, but he gave an impression of being larger than his missionary role. Later he lectured at the University of Saskatchewan, receiving a B.A. and an M.A. in 1912. He spent nineteen years in northern B.C., travelling around, measuring depths of lakes and talking with Indians about what it was like before the white man came. Instead of deciding that all their tribal rituals were primitive, he described them.

Later in my own travels I came across Father Maurice Metayer, another Oblate and, like Morice, far larger than the defined role. Their religion did not separate them from the people they lived with and they were not primarily concerned with gaining converts. Their seniors barely tolerated them at times. Unfortunately they were a minority in the sad history of colonial exploitation of Canada's north by religious zealots.

From Father Morice's book I learned of the Babines, the "Lippy People," whose women distended their lips with bone or wood. Then there were the Carrier and the Sekanais. I learned a great deal about these proud natives and where some of the various tribes might be located.

In Burns Lake we had a reserve. Amongst whites this reserve had a bad name because some of the Indians had drinking problems. Many felt horribly ashamed, so it took me some time to make friends with families on the reserve and to get them to talk. They are shy people and were, in those days, not used to whites trying to make social contact.

It took time to visit and learn the value of silence, after which some trust developed. No conversations would take place for quite a while, then some shared personal opinion about their kids would follow. After the barriers were broken, general conversation was easy.

Martha was an older Indian lady and a patient of mine.

She had chronic bronchitis and smoked too much. I would give her a bad time about smoking. I would also visit her at her home. One time I told her that if she gave up smoking, I would give up drinking. I of course said this just as a joke. On Tuesdays, a gang of us used to adjourn to the local pub, the Tweedsmuir Inn, after badminton. One Tuesday when I was in there drinking my twenty-five cent beer, Martha wandered over and said:

"White Man speaks with forked tongue."

I was caught out and she did not quit smoking, but always laughed at me over that. It seemed to give her some sort of edge over me, which made her more comfortable when I showed up for coffee at her house!

I learned about well known old families like "Kwah," modern spelling "Quah," who lived at Stuart Lake. There were bloody battles and the "Beavers" had "detonating bows," i.e. guns, which inflicted heavy damage on the Sekanais.

The white exploration went back a long way around here, with names such as Stuart and Fraser prominent. In 1806 Fraser was at Stuart Lake, east of then unnamed Burns Lake. Blais was over at Fraser Lake and the area known as New Caledonia. The Indians lived, for the most part, at Babine Lake, Francois Lake, Cheslatta and Ootsa Lake. At Old Fort Babine a Hudson's Bay post was established in 1822. It stands at the end of the lake in a most beautiful setting. I have flown around there many times in the Citabria looking for wolves, and have often landed on the ice near the old settlement.

My Citabria arrived in late 1971. I had been down to Vancouver and flown in it, but the day that it originally arrived in Burns Lake was an incredible thrill. I was at work in the clinic when I heard it over town. It was delivered by Jack Reilly, a former military pilot, now a dentist. The rest of the clinic staff followed me outside and then told me to get lost; they would sort out the clinic for that day! I shot out to the airport and then flew with Jack to Prince George. It was close to evening when I left Prince George and I merrily flew off in the wrong direction! I was so excited at my first solo in my own plane that I forgot to look at the compass. Soon it began to get dark. I had to return to Prince George and land there, after which I was called up to the tower to explain my antics. They were most understanding as it was my own new plane and next morning I made it back to Burns Lake via Vanderhoof, the right way.

Sir James Douglas, well known in later B.C. history, spent some time in his younger years at Fort St. James and was nearly killed by Kwah one day. I flew up, one winter day, to the area where that happened.

Sometime that same winter I met and fell in love with Judy, who had come to Burns Lake to work as a public health nurse. Judy loved to fly, and we had many flying adventures, subsequently marrying and moving up to the Arctic together.

The Citabria was, by this time, on skis. On a winter's morning we headed up Stuart Lake to Takla Landing, near Old Bulkley House. Judy and I were planning to do some ice-fishing. Only the bay was frozen, but there were skidoo tracks and snowshoe tracks and it looked safe. However just after touch down on the early fall ice, we broke through.

I probably touched down on land initially, on a point, and then, as I turned in towards a house belonging to local Indians, I noticed the inhabitants waving at me frantically. At about that moment Judy shouted to me that water was coming over the skis at the back. I hit full power but it was too late to take off; the suction was too great. We headed in to shore and made it by water skiing. The engine temperature was almost redlined by then. Closer to the shore the ice was more solid and held us. The take off, after a calming coffee break, was not a problem.

Peter Skene Ogden entered this area in 1834 and managed Hudson's Bay posts down as far as Kamloops (Fort Thompson). By 1844, the first missionaries were in the area. Most of them were "soul-catchers" and legacies, such as the lack of any rational Catholic birth control policy had, in general, quite a harmful influence. I would get a visit from some Indian lady who wanted to know if I could stop her having any more babies. I would discuss a tubal ligation. Some days later she would came back and say nothing when I asked her if she had decided. Then I would ask her what was going on; she would say that the priest told her it was wrong and a sin.

Some of the old Catholic schools were horrendous places. Nowadays we have all heard horror stories but I am sure Fr. Lejacq, a priest from the 1870 period, would have turned in his grave if he had seen how his school turned out. Through some delightful children, Rosie, Dennis, Randy and Corrina, I met their mother, Tina Jack. She had been to Lejacq school and told me many stories of the cruelty of the nuns.

For me, knowing some of this history helped to bring the area alive. Both the whites and the Indians gave me a sense of humility about the vastness and a feeling for the mysteries of the past. I started to read more about the far north and wanted to see it, but first I had to learn to fly better and improve my medical skills. From Doug Mann and George Magee in Burns Lake, I learned how to become a rounded family doctor and started to feel some confidence in a broad array of medical topics. I felt terribly inadequate surgically and wished I had known, when in training, what I would be doing three years after.

MAY 31, 1971: *Finished license on April 27th after 35.7 hours and did a flight test with Jack Lingham from the DOT. Then started right away on a float rating with Doug Tweedy in a Super Cub belonging to Trans Provincial. I teach him guitar, he teaches me floats. Trans Provincial think the plane is on a test flight. Today is a day off and I am at the float base by 9 a.m. Do an hour before lunch and then I have to go and do an anaesthetic; then back for an hour with Bill Harrison, a high time bush pilot. I do OK but do most of one circuit with the flaps still down and he punches me in the back and curses me. I don't do that again.*

Later that evening: off to the Canoe club, finishing up a canoe with help from Dave Foster and Martin Hobbs and other friends.

JULY 31ST—SATURDAY: *very busy—7-9.30 a.m. delivery with forceps. 9.30-11.30 anaesthetics for an emergency. Then I have to inject an IVP, do a barium meal X-Ray for an ulcer, do some suturing, followed by a quick lunch. After that over to the clinic down town and busy to make up for morning. Run, run, run but lots of fun!*

Most of the latter part of 1971 was spent learning practical medicine and building up to 90 hours of flying on the Citabria.

FEB. 1972: *Just pronounced silently inside my mind, the death sentence on a fourteen year old girl. She has a Rhabdomyosarcoma, a rare tumour inside her mouth and there is no more we can do for her. The family want me to tell them how long she will live. I have seen the secondaries on X-Ray, I say perhaps one year.*

She died within six months. I did not think I would ever get better at dealing with death and often wondered if other doctors found it as hard. I think we just did not talk about it much with each other. To talk about it, would probably have made it harder to deal with, not easier.

MARCH 1972: *A mysterious place, Burns Lake, with its fairy tale houses and gateways beyond to fields, little brooks and the unending forests. To me it offers adventures. Other houses hide behind mountains and skies of varying colour; the people seem almost slow, instinctive and accepting of the sense and pulse of nature. Myself, I am forever learning from them. The Indians here too are a part of this mystery, extending it backwards in time. They seem totally irrational in ways, yet deep and in touch with nature in others. In some there is a noble beauty and strength; this seems more evident in the women.*

Old Zennie Joseph is in her seventies with advanced bowel disease. She perforates her lower bowel, which causes an omental mass to seal it off. She walks out of the hospital saying she is going to the Indian doctor. Comes back the next day almost moribund. She pulls out the IV's we started and says nothing. I suspect the shaman told her she was going to die, so then she decided to return to us and die in the hospital.

At the clinic one well known local alcoholic is having a feigned epileptic seizure on the waiting room floor. He is thrashing around on the floor and threatening me with various consequences because I had not given him some narcotics he wanted. I am taken in by it but my partner, Doug Mann, comes in to the waiting room and threatens to kick him in the nuts unless he stops immediately. He adds that the RCMP will arrive as well. This arrests the farce. An overweight Indian lady sitting on the side, turns to all and sundry and says:

"Sure wish Dr. Mann would come and talk to my old man like that."

Andy George, also known as "Snoosebum," weighed 300 pounds and spent his life wandering between Smithers and Burns Lake. Mostly he hitch-hiked. He was banned for life from bars, due to the unfortunate early demise of two innocents who crossed him the wrong way. One was reputedly dropped from several feet on his head, then died a few weeks later but manslaughter was discarded. I don't know what happened to the other poor fellow. Andy was of sub-normal intelligence, and this, combined with an unpredictable nature, usually got him what he wanted when he came to see me. At the clinic, the other three members of the staff laughed at my early encounters with such characters and happily put them in with me. Andy took up most of the examining room. I would squeeze into the remaining space:

"What would you like today Andy?"

" 292's"

"How many?"

" 500!"

He would take these for his digestion, according to him.

He took two with every meal. It appeared prudent to meet his demands but we settled on two hundred and he departed happy. Doug and Joan, his wife and our nurse/assistant, and Joanne Crosbie, our "man Friday" inquired politely at coffee:

"Well how did you get on with old snoosebum?"

"Oh I gave him what he wanted, more or less."

"Very wise," they all commented, looking distinctly amused.

In March of 1972, I was taking another new doctor who had joined George Magee's practice, Dr. Ron Rushforth, up for a ride in the plane. It was getting late in the day and we were using a makeshift ice strip on Burns Lake. I showed him some loops and rolls but tended to snap roll less violently than normally, as I feared for the skis. As we landed on the thin packed ice strip, a crosswind drifted me off sideways. One ski caught in slush. I could not keep it straight so I tried to turn a complete circle with speed. Just then I got that sinking feeling and we broke through into water. We were not right through and the plane stayed up but Ron was cursing as this was his first flight.

I asked him to jump for it through the deep slush to the drier stuff. We walked through moderate slush to the shore. This was all within view of several friends, so, after a warm-up beer ashore, ten or so volunteers assembled.

It was now dark and quite cold. We put plywood under the skis; I sat inside and started the engine. Some of the helpers pushed on the wing struts and, as soon as the plane had skidded up onto the plywood, everyone got out of the way. I opened the throttle and booted for shore through the slush. The plane was fine. I thought everyone was in OK, so we all headed to the bar, where I had to buy of course! About thirty minutes later an annoyed Ron Rushforth arrived. He had been slugging in through the slush and no one realized that he was still out there. He did not appreciate the general laughter. He had been thinking of taking up flying, but for some reason he never did after this.

DEC. 1972: *Up at the hospital an old man of seventy was going through a somewhat painful death. He was a Caucasian and deserted by all his relatives, who could not deal with his dying. His eyes seemed to be asking me a question, yet he was unable to talk, because of his disease. I asked him everything I could think of until finally I asked him if he was afraid to die. That elicited a response. I talked of death and let him know that he would die soon. On hearing this he relaxed and I realized that he did not know he was dying. After I explained this to him he held my hand and soon passed away. I went home and listened to Bach's Toccata and Fugue in D minor, sitting alone in the dark, wondering how I would face my own death.*

Outside the house next morning there sat a woodpecker, busily eating away. I wanted to ask him where he was during the last three days, as it was below -50° F all the time.

On Christmas day the house heating system packed in. Outside, the temperature was -56° F. I called the Esso dealer and he came over and told me that I had lots of oil. It was frozen in the line. We had to "Tiger torch" the line, then lag it for insulation, and then I had heating again. In February my old friend, Adrian Cottrill from England, came over and we flew around, in the Citabria, on skis. We also drove one day, in my old Dodge Dart, down to Francois Lake at -55° F. It hurts the lungs to breathe too quickly when out walking around at that temperature.

SPRING 1973. SEASON CONTRAST: *Winter: cold, crisp, a time to turn into oneself. Plane on skis; battle with slush and deep snow. Clear calm flying, sometimes up to Noranda Mine at Babine Lake for clinics. Nice break in routine and so beautiful up by Babine in winter; landing up by the mine on the frozen lake. Then to summer and now 120° F hotter than in the cold spell. The country has come alive with colour. Green trees freshen the valley opposite my house. There are smells, forgotten since last year, brought out by the warmer weather. From the road below comes the noise of traffic, of dogs playing and panting in the sun. All these noises were not present in the silence of winter, broken only by the sorrowful, distant train whistle.*

Swallows glide around and one lone eagle, master of the sky, circles. He comes and checks me out when I fly near his territory; passed right by my wing once when I was upside down in a loop. The lake beneath me, when I fly, is glassy; not a breath of wind. Not even a boat down there today. It is a lazy summer day and in this season we get lazy and hedonistic, the winter forces us to be that way.

Chapter 4

ROSIE'S FAMILY

I came to know one nearby native family quite well, before I married. I cannot remember how it came about but they brought me great joy. They were to remain an important part of my life for many years and I came to love them all dearly.

Rosie, Corrina, Randy and Dennis had been wandering around my yard, playing, I seem to remember. I asked them if they would like to keep an eye on my place when I wasn't around. Later, they cleaned the house, fed my dog and looked after things when I was away. Rosie, who was about 12 or 13 at the time, was the oldest, and Corrina was 9, Randy 8 and Dennis 5 years old. They looked after everything for two years. Sometimes Rosie would have a cooked supper ready for me when I got home. Even the yard would be cleaned up. They had the keys to the house and were completely trustworthy. I was able to supplement their family income a little. Through these children and their mother, Tina Jack, I learned much about what it was like to be native.

They were non-status Indians, which meant they could not live on the reserve and were perhaps even more disadvantaged than the reserve Indians. I could visit them, but their world was quite different from mine and I did not want to be an intruder. Nor did I want to patronize them or manage their lives, so we became friends, especially Rosie and I. It was a friendship which lasted well into their adulthood, beyond Tina's death. I watched Randy go through all the tragic modern problems of alcohol, a criminal record and jail.

I talked at great length in later years with Rosie when she was suicidal, and I tried to give her some reason to battle on, in a very trying world for a young Indian woman. Shortly after I left Burns Lake, their mother had another child, Sabrina, and I became a kind of godfather to her. She was quite spoiled by the whole family and once took me very literally. I promised that she could come and visit me in 100 Mile House. One day in 1981, when visiting Burns Lake, I said to Sabrina:

"Well, Sabrina, you'd better get packed; we'll be off to 100 Mile House soon!"

I told her it was a long journey and was laughing while I said this. Then I left shortly after. Several months later, Rosie phoned me and could hardly stop laughing on the phone. She told me to talk to Sabrina, who was really mad with me. Poor Sabrina, who was around seven years old at the time, had packed her little bag and put in two loaves of bread for the journey. She had then placed the bag under her bed and patiently waited for me to come and fetch her. After three months she tearfully told Rosie that it did not look like I was going to come and she might as well unpack. They found the mouldy bread, twice the normal size! Sabrina was quite disgusted with me, the more so for all the laughter she had to endure.

Rosie was born in Burns Lake. Her ancestors came from Grassy Plains, across Francois Lake, towards Tweedsmuir Park. Her father was a reserve Indian, but Tina, Rosie's mother, had been a non-status for a long time, due to her association by marriage with a white man. Rosie lived with her grandma, Elsie Jack, for the first five years of her life, as her mother was into serious drinking. After Rosie moved back with her mom, things improved for a short time; then her mother began boozing again. When Randy was two and a half years old, Tina was saved from freezing to death. The newspaper boy found her in the snowbank, when doing his delivery. He notified the children that their mother was out there and helped them to bring her inside. She had locked the kids in the house and gone drinking.

Rosie learned to cook meals by the time she was six years old. Tina spent most days in the bar. Rosie would wake herself up, get meals for the younger kids, go to school and then come home and watch over her brother and sister. Some other relative would watch during the day. Rosie told me this story:

"Once, when Corrina was a baby, she wet herself and was crying. I didn't know she was wet and mom had come in drunk again. She went to check Corrina and told me to change her. I poked Corrina accidentally in the belly and mom got mad. She got a six foot two-by-four and started beating on me so I crawled under the stove and stayed there until she passed out. Randy was crying in sobs, asking mom to quit. Just about every night, when she came home, she took out her frustrations on me."

On one occasion, when Rosie was seven, Corrina asked her mom if they could drink some of the stuff in the fridge. There happened to be some pre-mixed whisky and pop, so all the kids got drunk. Their mom still drank fairly steadily when I first got to know them, but improved with time and quit altogether when Rosie was sixteen. She died not long after that. I kept trying to get Rosie more interested in getting educated as I saw that as the only hope for change within the native culture and for her own self image.

Rosie went through her own drinking time but became, later, a wonderful mother and our friendship has stayed until the present. Her mother wrote to me once, when I was working in Toronto, and asked me for help in dealing with Rosie's drinking problem. By this time Randy had been "inside" several times for breaking and entering. Rosie wrote to me about a painful time when one of her closest friends had committed suicide. In her letter she listed twenty-three of her friends and close relatives who had died violent deaths over the years. She even came to Toronto to visit at that time, but by then the essential differences of background and race were making it harder for me to help her anymore. My heart ached for the struggle she put up, trying so hard just to have a simple life without tragedies.

Through all these events they remained a close and amazingly happy bunch. When my own turn came to suffer some emotional turmoil, after some time in the Arctic, they accepted, without probing questions, that I just needed time to be there and rest up.

Rosie mentioned another story, which came from her Grandma, Elsie Jack. Rosie recorded it verbatim:

"Told to me by the elders of the past, it may be funny in parts, but it is as true as love can be. This story was told to my great-great-grandpa and he told it to his son, and he to his son and eventually it came to me, the great-great-great-granddaughter. The first grandpa he travelled all over the world. Long time ago he went to visit a tribe on the other side of the North Pole. These people were isolated and hardly anyone knew about them."

"He went to stay overnight, and just then a lady was having a baby and they didn't know how to give birth. The old ladies were sharpening knives and so were the men. Grandpa asked what they were up to. The father of the lady giving birth said they were going to cut her open to get the baby out. So grandpa told them they were going about it the wrong way. He told the woman to lean over a log and she did. He told the other woman to push down over her stomach and the baby came out and the woman lived. They were all so happy they started to cry. They all had small mouths and all they could eat were worms. They would kill prey and then let it rot until the worms came out, then eat."

"Now grandpa had a normal mouth, and one teenager asked him if he could have one too. They left the camp and went into the bush and grandpa cut slits to make his mouth larger. Then grandpa put pitch gum on it so it would heal fast. They went back to the tribe and they were all surprised and wanted the same. Grandpa spent three days cutting their mouths. This is one of our many happenings in our native life. This is what was told to me."

Corrina and Rosie have both settled, married and overcome many problems and had children. Sabrina has had more problems as her mom died when she was still quite young. For the boys it was so much harder. Randy had no way in which to prove his worth. The Indian male has had his masculinity questioned and his ability to go out and shoot a moose does not impress his dates anymore. His rites of adulthood are indefinite and he suffers from what Durckheim called 'anomie.' He resorts to drinking, suicide and drugs. Not truly a criminal, Randy spent many useless years in our jails. There his behaviour was reinforced and the path was downhill. This problem still remains unsolved for so many young native men, and one can only hope that education will ultimately help to solve it.

Chapter 5

FLYING TO ALASKA

In 1972, I made some practice flights to do medical clinics at Houston, about twenty minutes flying time from Burns Lake, and I landed in Gerald Baggerman's field with Joanne Crosbie, as my "nurse-assistant." By now I figured that I was ready for some serious flying. I trained early in the year for airshows, then volunteered for my first one at Dawson Creek in May. I used the parallel water runway to help align the aerobatics and it seemed to be OK. My airshow routine had been practiced over Burns Lake runway and consisted of basic rolls and loops, immelmanns, hammerheads, a snap roll at the top of a loop and then a clover leaf loop.

Later that summer, when I had built to the grand total of 165 hours, I performed at the Vanderhoof airshow, following which I was invited to participate in the Terrace airshow. At the Terrace show there were many professionals. Cliff Howard and his 'T-Minus-2,' a 180 HP Taylorcraft, was there, as were Howie Keefe and "Miss America," and Skip Volk. Skip flew a modified De Havilland Chipmunk. Ormond Haydon-Baillie had his Hawker Sea Fury.

Included in Cliff Howard's show was an inverted ribbon cutting act; I held the poles for the ribbon. That is when you really trust the pilot! Pat Johnston was flying his Citabria and I booked some aerobatic time with him for later in the year, as he was an excellent performer. Sad to say, he died in the Prince George airshow one week later.

Most of the participants in this show were killed in flying accidents within a few years, including Haydon-Baillie who advised me that I needed to practice more if I were going to do airshows. I had misjudged my recovery height from a loop and clipped a few branches at one end of the runway. Normally I did not go below 400 feet, so my error was over 200 feet. I decided to stay alive and quit doing airshows until I could afford more time for practice.

Later that year, I decided that I had enough hours to head off into the wild blue yonder, with Judy. We planned to go to Alaska. On August 14th, we departed from Burns Lake. The Citabria was loaded from floor to ceiling in the baggage area. I had flown 175 hours in twelve months, a lot for a private pilot, so I felt confident though apprehensive. We headed over to Mackenzie via Fort St. James, and enroute talked with the pilot of a Bonanza who had lost a bit of his propeller, but was still able to fly. He made it in to Prince George, complaining of major vibration, but there was nowhere to land until he cleared the mountains.

We camped overnight at Chetwynd and then went over to the Pruckl Farm. I had met the owner at an airshow, earlier in the year. He had said to come by, so we landed on his primitive grass strip and had breakfast with him and his family. We then headed on over to Fort Nelson for gas, but decided to detour to the "Headless Valley," better known as the South Nahanni River. We landed at Nahanni Butte, camped for a few days and also met up with Don Turner. Unfortunately we were not able to cross the river to meet his father, Dick, who later wrote "Wings of the North." At Nahanni, I traded some gas for an aerobatic display, which meant unloading the whole plane. By then we needed to shovel out dead blackflies and mosquitoes anyway!

When Judy and I took off later, there were so many bugs that we went up to 12,000 ft. Up there they went to sleep for a while, but as soon as we descended they woke up again! Whilst at Nahanni, I had to do a mercy mission for some doctors and dentists out of Dawson Creek. This involved a trip to Ft. Nelson for some spare engine parts for their boat. They had come down the South Nahanni. On the way back from Ft. Nelson a lightning bolt went down right ahead of me, just missing the plane. I had turned off all radios as I had seen the proximity of the storm.

Back at Nahanni, I discovered a little Ercoupe parked right up in the trees. Some middle aged lady pilot had some trouble with carburettor icing and had to put down at Nahanni, but missed the airstrip and popped it into the trees. She was not hurt but was quite annoyed that nobody had seen her, and that she had to wait a long time before anyone came to her assistance.

Leaving Nahanni on August 19th we encountered lousy weather; fog and rain, so we scooted low level to Fort Liard. There we saw the boat belonging to the group we had helped out; they treated us to a good steak lunch. Afterwards the weather lifted and we headed for Liard River. This was one of the wartime strips built to help deliver planes to Russia, and to assist with the construction of the Alaska highway.

We landed and parked at one end, on the grass, and looked down the length of this deserted 6000' grass runway. It was so peaceful there. We started to cook supper and a lone wolf wandered across the runway. Towards evening an excitable Quebecois, who flew in with a small Piper, joined us. An American couple arrived shortly after, in a Cessna 170, with crosswind landing gear. We all shared supper, had a sing-song, then all flew the next day to Whitehorse. The airport there was not that busy in those days and we were the only planes going north. When we were in town shopping someone came up to us and said:

"Are you the owners of that blue and white Citabria parked by the helicopters?"

We did not know that some US military Chinooks had arrived. The downblast had damaged some planes near us but had spun mine around on the tiedown. Luckily there was no damage. I was quite upset at the helicopter pilot. We left Whitehorse and flew on to the Alaskan border, crossing at Northway, after a detour to Atlin. The customs officer thought that I had hashish on board. I kept telling him it was pipe tobacco but he saw my guitar and made me empty the plane. Later he took us to lunch as he felt badly. After lunch we heard that a plane was overdue and volunteered to go and look, as nobody else was ready. The missing pilot was in a Smith Miniplane and after 20 minutes we saw him, out by the edge of the mountains. He was still flying, but low on gas and had a good place picked out to land and refuel. We relayed all this back to Flight Service and everyone was happy. We were happy he was safe in those forbidding mountains. There is great camaraderie amongst pilots facing the same challenges.

We were in Fairbanks by August 24th; then we headed west, trying for the Bering Sea. Unfortunately bad weather forced us in to Manley Hot Springs, where we had to pay for drinking water, and camp in the rain. After a couple of days we changed direction and went back to Fairbanks to dry out. Then we headed south to Summit, where we camped and took buses up into Denali Park; plenty of Grizzly Bears to see there! We decided to go and take pictures of the summit of Mt. McKinley—after all we did have a plane! We climbed up to 14,500', slightly short of breath, due to the altitude, and took some pictures. By then I was above an almost solid cloud layer and got disoriented.

Flying above clouds is legal in the United States for pilots under VFR or Visual Flight Rules, but not in Canada, so we were legal. I was able to get a glimpse of a glacier through a hole in the clouds, and followed the advice I had read in an Alaskan book. I did have a radial off one VOR, a pilot's navigation device. VOR stands for VHF Omnirange. The book had said all glaciers lead down to rivers which, in turn, lead out to the sea through valleys. That was where we wanted to go and sure enough the glacier came out north of Anchorage.

By September 3rd, we were back in Whitehorse and decided to head through Carcross to Atlin. Here we met Herman Pederson, a well known old bush pilot. He cautioned us about flying over the Taku Inlet to get to Juneau, but that was the way we flew. We had a solid cloud cover right past Juneau. Some careful calculation and compass flying would have worked out except for the tailwind at 12,000 ft. I finally found a hole out over the ocean and descended to a cloud base of 2500' over an ocean of icebergs. This did not look friendly but the good news was that we were closer to Juneau than to Japan! We made it in to Juneau in light rain and waited for an improvement in the weather.

Later that day, the weather report looked good all the way to Prince Rupert, so we headed off. Sad to say, the weather can be most inhospitable up there, and by the time we had reached Annette Island, north of Rupert, it socked in. We had to map read down to 500 feet, and go in to Wrangell for the night. The rest of the trip home was uneventful and by then I had reached almost 300 hours in two years of flying.

That winter I put on another 70 hours of ski flying. There was some excitement on a flight to Babine Lake, with Lutz Boeker from Burns Lake. We had gone for a sightseeing trip and the ice looked good where I touched down, but we hit a spot where a river came in and we broke through into slush. The cylinder head temperature was close to redline as we headed straight for an open ferry crossing at Granisle. Luckily we lifted off a few hundred yards short of the ferry crossing.

Doug Mann and I started the clinics at Houston. I flew, whenever possible, landing at Gerald Baggerman's field. Joanne Crosbie came along to help. Joanne knew that the medical bag was fastened tightly under the rear seat and that the short flight over to Houston would involve some aerobatics. Gerald Baggerman Sr. was a kindly old man. He and his wife were always most hospitable to me. He just loved planes and had two airstrips at 90 degrees, both grass of course. On the approach to one you would come in over trees, pull full flaps just over the trees to steepen the approach, then point the plane quickly to the ground and add a little power to soften the touchdown. The other runway was easier. Mrs. Baggerman always put tea on, to settle our stomachs after our aerobatics.

In Burns Lake, in spite of the warning from the College of Physicians, I found the doctors and nurses taught me a great deal about medicine. They had to be resourceful because of the isolation. At that time Air Ambulances were not developed at all. From the old pioneers I learned much about the Burns Lake traditions and the old established families. They made great patients and were most appreciative of a new doctor.

Our hospital was often filled to capacity; beds would be in the corridor, sometimes as many as ten extra beds. At times, three doctors would look after over fifty in-patients. Many Indian children had severe otitis media or respiratory infections during the first few years of their life. Scabies was rampant, until public health improved. We were forced to admit some of the small children for weeks on end. If alcohol was a factor in the family, keeping the child for a while was a good idea and it might clear up the scabies, commonly present all over the scalp and the face. Cases of meningitis were quite common. We admitted them, started scalp vein infusions and loaded them up with antibiotics. I was thankful I had done some paediatrics before coming here.

MAY 1973: *The Lakes District is a deceptive area. Like many northern towns, the town itself is unremarkable, yet it becomes the centre for all sorts of exploration of a beautiful region. I escape by road as well as by plane, to magic places like Tchesinkut Lake, Francois Lake, Grassy Plains, Ootsa Lake. Beyond that lies Tweedsmuir Park and to the north Babine Lake. There is never enough time to see it all. Flying over Mt. Wells, in Tweedsmuir Park, I filmed a herd of 60-70 caribou up in the deep snow, last winter. In the summer I took trips in the "Jacob Henkel," the Francois Lake ferry, and took a step back in time. Burns Lake is not exactly fast paced city living, but Grassy Plains was another century!*

By 1973, Judy and I decided to move along. I was quite happy in Burns and had my friends and my plane, but Judy wanted to see a little more of the world so we decided to sell my beloved Citabria and I found a job in Nigeria.

On June 15th, I flew what would turn out to be my last aerobatics flight for a while, and gave Mr. Baggerman a private airshow.

.... Took off, climbed steeply with two notches of flap at 60 mph. Levelled off at 1500', up with the flaps and got 120 mph and full power. Vertical stall to the right; recovered; added power to increase airspeed to 140 mph and pulled back over in a loop. Pulled a little "G" on the recovery. Climbed again and slowed to 70, then hit the rudder and full back stick, careful as she went round in a snap roll, recovering a bit late as usual. Now 145 mph, then a loop and, at the top, whilst inverted, did the snap roll and recovered inverted. Followed up with some split-s manoeuvres from half-snaps, then, from a higher altitude, a few turns of a spin and back to the ground—touched the wheels on the runway at 120 mph—then vertical to 700 agl. Power dive back down and touched one wheel only on the runway. Steep, fast turn, then popped the flaps on, got the speed down to 75 mph and crept over the fence for a downwind landing—running up close to the house before parking the plane..........

We sold the Citabria to a local resident. I tied her down feeling sad. Life in Burns Lake had been quite idyllic for me and the plane was a symbol of the freedom which I had felt.

Judy and I flew to England, from where we intended to drive down through the Sahara Desert to Nigeria. Purchasing a Volkswagen camper for this purpose, we ventured around Europe to kill some time. In the meantime, however, the Nigerian Government, decided that they needed a black doctor. We had to decide whether to start looking for jobs in that part of the world or return to Canada. My desire to get to the Arctic prevailed and Judy agreed to return to Canada and to go together to the Arctic. We booked immediately on the "Stefan Batory," a Polish Lines Atlantic ship, and headed back to Montreal and Ottawa.

Chapter 6

THE ARCTIC BECKONS

There is a certain fascination, or perhaps we can even say disease, which affects many who read stories of polar exploration. What is it? A desire for the purity of the frozen wastes; a certain longing for open spaces? The Greeks believed in a land called after the north wind (Boreas), where Hyperboreans lived in peace and harmony, in a land of perpetual sunshine. Well perhaps this is it—in the summer!

Some who fall in love with the north are sad escapees from some insoluble turmoil inside themselves. There is a certain paranoia, and also misanthropy, in many northerners. A number of plain misfits and real characters end up heading for the Arctic. I was somewhere in the middle of all of this; somewhere between turmoil and curiosity and desire for adventure.

But what lured all these explorers to the north? Just the Northwest Passage? It had to be more; this 'Polar Passion' had to be more complex. I was developing it long before I went north. Perhaps, ultimately, it was the personal challenge, to overcome inner fears and be able to live with oneself. Think of John Hornby, that very strange Englishman, who died such a pointless death out on the barrens! He went north time and time again, with ill-prepared trips; almost a suicidal element to them; until finally he succumbed to the winter and died of starvation.

As for myself, I was curious and definitely a misfit. I sought a place where I could both be a doctor and have time to read more of my precious philosophy. I was infected with the Arctic 'bug'. I studied the history and ultimately ended up doing a degree in Northern Studies. Even now, years after leaving the north, excited meetings take place with other ex-northerners. Politics of self-determination, native rights and mineral exploration are all discussed. It is as if we were still involved over twenty years later. For various reasons we choose not to live in the Arctic anymore, but we miss the intensity.

During my last months in Burns Lake I began reading about the north. Whilst killing time in the U.K., we earned gliding licenses and I read Vilhjalmur Stefansson's 'The Friendly Arctic.' This was his account of his travels during the First World War, as part of the Canadian Arctic Expedition. It is a controversial book; many who read it do not agree that the Arctic is that friendly. However, he achieved much himself, and also interested many people in the north and in their ability to conquer their fears of the environment. He certainly got me hooked.

I knew that I would have to go and see this place for myself. At that time I felt that it was going to be, for me, essentially an inner journey. I was obviously seeking something inside myself, but I did not know exactly what. I was lucky enough to be in a job where I could travel in the Arctic; see Canada's last true frontier and get paid for it. The isolation would have a harmful effect on my medical knowledge, as it would be very different medicine up there, but I was not aware of that at the time. The history excited me so much that I really did not mind where I went, as long as it was in the true Arctic.

In Montreal, after the boat crossing of the Atlantic, we purchased a Volkswagen to drive back to British Columbia. We stopped in Ottawa, to meet up with Dr. Lyle Black at Medical Services for Northern Health. It seemed that I would have to wait, but not for long. We headed on to B.C. and I read more and more about the Arctic.

My reading gave me a feeling of living history, just as I had felt in Burns Lake. Only a few years had passed since the last group of Inuit moved into permanent housing. Within memory of those still living, Amundsen had traversed the Northwest Passage. Rasmussen and Stefansson had been up there travelling, and had made some of the first ever contacts with Inuit tribes. Here were places I could go and speak to people who might even remember these famous explorers, but, more importantly, I could see the areas first hand.

I read everything I could get my hands on, including Samuel Hearne's record of his expedition with Matonabbee from Churchill to Coppermine. Here, in 1771, Hearne had to sit and watch while Matonabbee and his crew massacred a whole group of Inuit at Bloody Falls. In 1789, while the Revolution was starting in France, Alexander Mackenzie trekked through to Whale Island, at the mouth of the river now bearing his name. Four years later, he completed the first crossing of the continent, north of Mexico, and reached the Pacific Ocean at Bella Coola. By this time the British knew that any passage to the Indies had to go north of the Mackenzie and the Coppermine rivers, and stay north of Hudson Bay.

Why not go straight across the Polar Sea? It was thought that there would be open sea somewhere up there; a belief that persisted for a long time. Many famous sailors put in their apprenticeship in the Arctic, Horatio Nelson being one. At age fifteen, Nelson was on a ship called the 'Carcass'. He served under Captain Lutwidge and nearly lost his life when hunting a polar bear. He missed with his musket and narrowly made it back to the ship followed by an angry bear.

Money entered the picture when the Council of the Royal Society of London offered £20,000 to anyone passing through the Northwest Passage. Captain Cook had this ambition and sailed through the Bering Straits in 1778, and made it to Icy Cape, at latitude 70°, before being turned back by ice. Then he journeyed on to Unalaska and his fate in Kauai, in the Hawaiian Islands.

Following this era, a new, more realistic image of the passage emerged; that of the ice-filled route among barren lands. New explorations, pushed by Sir John Barrow headed into the area. William Scoresby Jr., a whaler of note, continued to entertain the idea of an open Polar Sea. There began a famous period of exploration. In 1818, Sir John Ross with Lieutenants W.E. Parry, John Franklin and George Back, took off with four ships on an ambitious trip. Two ships headed north to try for the Polar Sea; the other two were to find, and sail through, the Northwest Passage. James Ross was a midshipman on his uncle's ship and harpooned a whale for them when they reached the Greenland coast. They met the Etah Eskimos, later famous for helping Peary reach the Pole. John Ross sailed into Baffin Bay as far as Lancaster Sound, but thought that there was no way through and turned back. This conclusion caused his disgrace as further persistence would have shown that there was a passage through to the west.

Parry, in the second ship did not see land at the end of the sound. In contrast to Ross, he believed that it was possible to traverse that way. Later he was proved to be correct. Ross was disgraced when he returned to England and the next year's expedition was led by Parry. He took the 'Hecla' and the 'Griper' and made it well into Lancaster Sound, naming Beechey Island and accomplishing the first ever winter stay by an explorer's ship. The sun disappeared on November 4th for ninety-six days. The ship did not move again until August 1st, with the first open water. The expedition made it back to England by November 3rd, 1819.

For the next forty years many names came up again and again, but of course one cannot fail to be intrigued by the Franklin drama. Sir John Franklin fascinated me as his name was so prominent in the Western Arctic. The last unexplored portion of the N.W. Passage was around Cambridge Bay, now called Ikaluktutiak. Franklin, on his second trip north in 1820-1822, made it as far as Point Turnagain, in Coronation Gulf, travelling along the coast, by land and with small canoes. This epic journey, which nearly ended in total tragedy, has been well documented in the diaries of Dr. John Richardson. The diary was edited and published, as 'An Arctic Ordeal', by a radiologist in Saskatoon, Dr. Stuart Houston. He has had a long interest in the history and biology of that part of the Arctic, and in later years asked me to fly over part of Franklin's earlier route, to check for any remaining buildings from their trip.

The maps of that era show a vast gap from Point Turnagain, just south of Victoria Island, to the area around Resolute. Franklin returned for a third trip, in 1825. He went to New York, then to Great Bear Lake, and then, with two twenty-six foot boats, he explored 1200 miles of coastline. Richardson and Beechey accompanied him on this expedition. Whatever hindsight may have shown us about the reason why all Sir John Franklin's crew perished on his last expedition in 1845, hauling expensive silver etc., I have always felt a sense of awe about his earlier travels. This was reinforced by visiting those stretches of desolate coastline.

What a region to explore! When I traversed this area myself, in the seventies, by snowmobile and later by flying low along the entire coastline, I was left in total awe at the endurance and courage of the explorers. The two birchbark canoes weighed 300 lbs each and were set on two sledges fore and aft. Three or four men and two dogs helped to drag these over the snow.

In 1829, Sir John Ross entered the picture once more. Desperately seeking to mend his reputation, after being misled by the false appearance of a blocked Lancaster Sound, he was able to get financing now that Parry had retired. Felix Booth, of the well-known distillery, helped him out. Twenty-four men went along, including his nephew, James Ross. They set off to Lancaster Sound. This time they went in to where the 'Fury' lay wrecked, to refill their stores. During the winter, James Ross walked across the Boothia Peninsula to King William Island, almost to where Franklin had reached from the west. James Ross was also the first to locate the North Magnetic Pole. In 1974 I had the good fortune to make a snowmobile trek across that very same route.

James Ross now repeated the error of his uncle and reported no way through, by ship, east of King William Island. Mirages occur in areas like this. I was able to confirm this in that exact spot, where James Ross had crossed. Land masses appear to be visible in all directions. This was exciting to me, as they would have been the similar mirages which misled the early explorers. Sir John Ross and his nephew were among the first to appreciate that to prevent scurvy, fresh or even raw meat was necessary. This they learned from the locals. They had to abandon their ship and made it home after two winters to relative, albeit late, fame.

The remaining part of the Passage still to be explored and charted, was finished by land in a series of trips by Back, Dease, Simpson and John Rae, three of these being Hudson's Bay men.

In May of 1845, Sir John Franklin with his two ships, left the river Thames, on his fateful journey. At close to sixty, he set off on a trip that Sir James Ross himself, by then forty-five, believed he was too old to endure. Sir John Ross stated that they would all perish. Franklin had fought at the Battle of Trafalgar and had been Governor of Tasmania. He took the 'Erebus' and the 'Terror', with Captain Crozier as second-in-command. Nothing was heard from the expedition after 1845. By 1847, the most expensive and longest search in history began. It was to last almost ten years and cost millions of pounds. Sir John Ross, then over seventy, went back looking for Franklin.

McClure found a new route to explore the N.W. Passage, up the Prince of Wales Straits by Banks Island, but he failed to get right through. Indeed this route remains impassable most years, as it is almost always icebound. Captain Collinson, in the 'Enterprise', went as far as Cambridge Bay, wintering there in 1852-1853. At that time he was within sledging distance of the few remaining survivors of the Franklin expedition, but he had no way of knowing where they were.

The rescuers were forced to begin rescuing each other and many ships were left behind. Captain McClintock, with the 'Fox', sailed all around the area of the tragedy, and described the West Coast of King William Island as the most desolate place that he had ever seen. I agreed with him, many years later, when I flew a Maule M5-235 plane at low level from Cambridge Bay across the straits and across King William Island.

It remained for Dr. John Rae, a fur trader and physician with the Hudson's Bay Company, to send word of the apparent fate of the Franklin Expedition, north of the Back, or Fish, River. On September 28th, 1854, the sailors arrived back in England with some of the news. Rae had found relics on King William Island and also discovered the important passage to the south of King William Island. This southern route was ultimately Amundsen's, on his successful trip through the N.W. Passage.

In October of 1854, John Rae sent a letter to the Admiralty in London relating his findings. He had left Repulse Bay on this particular expedition. To the north-west, he had encountered Eskimos who told him stories of white men who had died from starvation. Rae obtained spoons, forks and other relics which left no doubt that these were from the Franklin ships. He claimed and received the £10,000 prize for determining the fate of the Franklin Expedition. Lady Franklin, Sir John's widow, was not satisfied and financed yet another expedition. Captain Leopold McClintock undertook a voyage with the 'Fox', during which he found documents. Gore and Fitzjames had written these last words and left them in cairns, on the desolate west coast of King William Island, before they had all starved to death.

Captain Kellet's own ship, 'Resolute', later drifted out of the ice on its own. The United States government refitted it and sent it back to the British. It is also possible that McClure's abandoned ship, the 'Investigator', drifted down past King William Island. Three years earlier, in 1851, a reliable sighting had been made of two ships drifting by Newfoundland. This gives strength to the theory that Franklin's ships were abandoned and drifted on their own into the Atlantic. Stories of Eskimo sightings to the west and south of King William Island may have been referring to the 'Investigator' and have fuelled many a search. Franklin himself had died, in 1847, shortly before the abandonment of his two ships. The search for wreckage from the ill-fated expedition continues until the present day. There is even a society set up to finance expeditions to find answers to this mystery.

I read about modern explorers as well. Henry Larsen's trip, in the years 1940-1944, through the Northwest Passage, would be within living memory of people whom I would meet. I did subsequently meet George Washington Porter, who had been a guide on Larsen's ship. George was an Inuit from Gjoa Haven.

Roald Amundsen, a Norwegian, probably lays claim to being the greatest polar explorer of all times. He was certainly the most successful, and planned all his expeditions meticulously. He did not believe in adventure and thought that if an expedition turned into an adventure, that it was from poor planning. In June of 1903, he left Norway, barely ahead of creditors, for a three year trip through the N.W. Passage. The 'Gjoa' was 72 feet long and had a beam of 11 feet. The first winter for the expedition was spent at what is now known as Gjoa Haven, and there Amundsen met up with the Eskimos. This would have been the first contact since their grandfathers had met Sir James Ross, seventy-two years earlier. According to Amundsen, the rest of his trip was almost routine, and he succeeded in being the first to sail through the Passage, after a long overland trek from Herschel Island for supplies.

The excitement of reading all this had me impatiently awaiting a call from Northern Health. In the meantime I accepted a temporary job in Whitehorse, to get us closer to the "true north."

Chapter 7

CAMBRIDGE BAY

In early 1974, Judy and I headed up the Alaska Highway in our old VW station wagon. This was definitely more dangerous than any flying I had done! The White Pass and Yukon trucks were intent on boring down the highway and did not seem inclined to slow down for anything. This meant that I lost visibility, due to the blowing dust, and drove blind for several hundred yards after they passed. In the meantime I tried to keep vaguely to the right, without going off the shoulder of the road. The stark beauty of the Yukon impressed us, but I was not too happy about being stuck in Whitehorse. I was impatient to go and see the Arctic.

Soon after we arrived in Whitehorse, we received an offer to go to Cambridge Bay, on the Central Arctic Coast. Should we stay longer in the Yukon? The answer came quickly. Most of my reading had been centred on the Western Arctic so I was happy to get the Central/Western Arctic. How long should we plan on being there? Dr. Otto Schaefer, in Edmonton, an old Arctic guru, suggested staying a couple of years to get a feel for the Inuit culture and language.

I stayed two and a half years in Cambridge Bay. The sociological pressures became harder as communications improved. It also became harder to get back into normal medicine when technology was changing so fast. There was extensive air travel and peer isolation. The department had recently become more cautious about any extra persons on flights, following the Hartwell crash out of Cambridge Bay. This meant that Judy would be stuck in Cambridge Bay a lot of the time on her own. Our marriage was not to survive the time in Cambridge Bay. This could not be blamed on the location, but it might have been an easier problem to deal with elsewhere.

Martin Hartwell, the pilot involved in the ill-fated flight, had responded to urgent pressure to fly some patients out of Cambridge Bay to Yellowknife, in early winter. The plane was a twin-engine Beech 18. On board were a nurse from Spence Bay and two Inuit patients; one pregnant lady and a young boy with appendicitis. Hartwell and the boy survived the crash. There was controversy over whether he should have declined the flight and let a later scheduled DC-3 take the patients. I imagine that there was considerable pressure on the pilot, something I witnessed many times. In fact, neither of these cases should have been such high priority. In that sense, it was a needless tragedy.

Hartwell had run into snow and was flying in IFR, or Instrument Flying Rules, conditions. He had tried to stay visual, but, due to poor reception from the Contwoyto Lake NDB, he went off course and crashed into low hills. An NDB is a Non-Directional Beacon, used by pilots for navigation.

The young Eskimo boy survived 23 days, so his appendicitis was presumably not too severe. Hartwell survived beyond Search and Rescue's estimates, with both ankles badly injured, until he was rescued after 30 days. Unfortunately, he was honest about his method of survival in the final days and the media made much of the cannibalism issue. He became a scapegoat for some wrong decisions, poor aircraft maintenance, and poor navigation aids. Many years later I got lost in good weather, using the same beacon. The popular versions of this tragedy failed to bring out the pilot's side of the story.

I arrived at Cambridge Bay shortly after this tragedy. My conclusion was that, in sending patients off in really bad weather, I would have to balance medical risks against aviation risks.

Talking over these things and many other aspects of northern medicine with Dr. Otto Schaefer, in Edmonton, was of inestimable value. At that time he was the Research Doctor with Northern Health and was based at the Charles Camsell Hospital. He had great affection for the Inuit and other northern natives he had worked with. He had served in Pangnirtung and Aklavik, was fluent in the language of the north, and was an inspiration to many of us younger doctors. The Camsell Hospital had a staff dedicated to looking after patients from the north, with as much cultural sensitivity as they could learn, and the patients felt at home there; as much as one can in a hospital.

From Edmonton Judy and I and our two dogs, Bushmills and Baggins, headed by PWA jet, up to Yellowknife. There I met several of the local physicians. They were a great source of strength to me when I was dealing with difficult cases, all alone. The Stanton Hospital, in Yellowknife, was 540 nautical miles south of Cambridge Bay. Edmonton was a further 550 miles and was the next referral centre. In Cambridge Bay, I would be based and live in that community. From there I would cover Gjoa Haven, Spence Bay and Pelly Bay to the east, and Bathurst Inlet, Bay Chimo, Coppermine and Holman Island to the west and south. I received no specific orientation from anyone other than Otto Schaefer, because nobody else at the Camsell had actually tried doing that kind of job. In response to my queries about clinics and visits to communities, they said to me:

"Go there and you'll see what is needed!"

I wanted to know if I was expected to do kitchen table appendectomies and was very glad to be told that I should fly them out! I had only ever performed a couple, in a normal hospital, and they were under supervision. They gave me no anaesthetic equipment and no supply of blood in Cambridge Bay. I began to hope that nobody was going to get seriously ill whilst I was up there. My only instructions about the job were that there were nurses in most of these communities, and I should "oversee" what they were doing; however, I had no mandate for any kind of administrative seniority over them. It all sounded rather vague; as if I were just going to be some kind of "presence."

The main village of Cambridge Bay had only been there for about 20 years—since the Dewline Station was built. First named in 1831 by Simpson and Dease, of the Hudson's Bay company, it had only received sporadic visits from whites. In 1851, John Rae was there on the Franklin search, then in 1852 Collinson with the 'HMS Enterprise'. He hiked the twelve miles in to Mt. Pelly, our only break in the totally flat land. Stefansson was there in 1910, and in 1921 the Hudson's Bay Company opened a store at Cambridge Bay. They used Amundsen's old boat the 'Bay Maud'. This had been used, unsuccessfully, by Amundsen as the 'Queen Maud', in his attempt to navigate the Northeast Passage during the First War. The company used it as a radio ship, and in 1929 transmitted a message that some well known explorers, thought lost, had turned up successfully in Cambridge Bay. These were the Dominion explorers who had flown from La Pas, Manitoba, to explore the Bathurst Inlet area.

Henry Larsen stayed there over part of World War II with the 'St. Roch', during his epic voyage through the Northwest Passage. After that period a settlement was established to the west of the existing one and the original Catholic church still stands there. Nearby are the remains of the 'Bay Maud', slightly under the surface of the sea. The church had been built in 1954 by Father LeMer. He used seal oil and sand and large stones to 'cement' the building. As the Dewline began, the village naturally moved across to the other side of the bay. The Dewline station was constructed in 1955 as part of the radar link across the north. Originally, radar stations were spaced every fifty miles. By the time I lived there every second station had closed. Now they are all left as a peculiar reminder of the paranoia of the times.

The stations were originally staffed by the United States Airforce, but by 1974 there were many more Canadian military officers there and gradually more civilians were hired for the day to day operations. Living on one of these Dewline Stations was like living in another world. Little contact was encouraged with either the village nearby, or reality itself, and the ultimate control was in Denver,

Colorado. The Cambridge Bay station was only three miles from the village, yet it seemed like visiting another planet when we went out there. This we willingly did, as the food was also out of this world to us deprived northerners!

Cambridge Bay sits on the pre-cambrian shield, with Mt. Pelly, at 600' in the background. It takes a few hours to hike to Mt. Pelly which is the only landmark for many, many miles. In January the average temperature is -30°F and the wind averages 15 mph. In the summer it occasionally warms up to 60°F. The sun sets for good in early December, to reappear after six or seven weeks. By April, one can travel and hunt in almost total daylight. Interestingly, the difficulty is adapting to the increased daylight, not to the few months of darkness. In winter everyone sleeps a lot; in the summer hardly at all. My first impression was that getting to know the Inuit was going to be fascinating. They seemed open and friendly and very curious about us.

The doctor was given a comfortable house and I never had problems getting furniture given to me. I just could not get any advice on the job! The nurses were in charge of the nursing stations and that left me in limbo!

Doctors came and went, most staying only a few months, so the nurses got used to running everything. Some did incredible work and managed well; others panicked over every case and used medevacs regularly. It was very hard for someone 1000 miles away to tell them that they did not need to send the patient out. For some of the nurses, it was an escape from working with doctors. Here the nurses could perform many things they would not be allowed to do in the south. Indeed most of the procedures were performed as well as they would be by any doctor, though penicillin tended to be over-prescribed for minor illnesses.

Isolation for the doctor was total; and even worse for one well versed in Canadian style medicine. In Medical Services, as soon as a doctor became "promoted," and moved to Yellowknife or Edmonton, he became a bureaucrat and lost touch with the realities of isolation medicine. The nurses, at least, had one another for some peer contact. I had my fellow doctors in Yellowknife, 540 miles and a three and a half hour flight away, in good weather. They were most supportive. They were however, not employees of the Federal Government and still lived in a more normal world. This meant that it was difficult for them to relate to the conditions under which we worked.

We were flown up to Cambridge Bay in a De Havilland Twin Otter—luggage, dogs, the lot. Judy and I were the only passengers. Somewhere north of Yellowknife we began to realize that we were now going to be a long way from anywhere. Yellowknife still seemed to be part of the 'world', but now we had crossed an invisible line on the earth's surface, demarcating a world with different rules. There would be no fresh milk for the next few years, eggs would not be shipped up here, butter came only in cans and there would be no such thing as fresh tomatoes or lettuce. Occasionally we might see onions. Coca Cola arrived in the Hudson's Bay store, priced lower than an apple. Pringles potato chips were in abundance. We had crossed a mystical line. I felt that the Arctic was not so much a geographical entity as a state of mind. The engines droned on as we crossed endless miles of snow covered tundra. It was to be the first of hundreds of hours spent sitting in Twin Otters.

As soon as I arrived at the airport at Cambridge Bay, I got an idea as to how the new doctor would be welcomed. To meet us, and carry us into town, was the sewage truck! The nurses had sent this, although they did have a four-wheel drive vehicle. They were making a point! There had been no doctor here for six months. I had been wasting my time in Whitehorse and they had told me there were no openings in the Arctic, yet there had been no doctor here for six months. Prior to that an old friend of mine, Dr. Carl Gill, had been up here and had stayed for one summer.

The nurses in Cambridge Bay itself were enjoying their freedom immensely and resented my arrival. My job description gave me authority for the Central Arctic area but not over any actual place! I was a visitor in all nursing stations, even in Cambridge Bay where I resided! I had ultimate medical authority over medevacs but no administrative power at all. As far as local nurses were concerned, I could only intervene if obvious medical mismanagement was taking place. I had to beg permission to use their vehicle so that my wife could fetch our groceries from the store or to go to the airport and meet the plane.

The Eskimos regarded me with respect, as a senior 'shaman', and one could also earn such respect by speaking, or attempting to speak, their language and hunting and travelling with them. The whites thought I ran the nursing station too. We did have in-patient facilities, but the nurses did not like to keep patients; they preferred to ship most of them south, even minor cases. This scenario applied only in Cambridge Bay; in the outlying stations the doctor was always welcomed and performed consultation clinics.

My 'practice' here covered a vast area. Spread across the central/western Arctic, it covered a distance, laterally, equivalent to that from Vancouver, British Columbia, to Regina, Saskatchewan! Three thousand inhabitants resided in the region, and communications were by air, snowmobile or boat. We were 540 nautical miles north of Yellowknife, the nearest inhabited town to the south.

I visited each outlying settlement a couple of times and then, disappointed with an evident lower standard of medicine in Cambridge Bay itself, began clinics at my home base. In the town itself we had 700 Inuit and maybe 100 whites, with another 50 at the Dewline. All the other communities were smaller, with few non-Inuit.

Soon after arriving at Cambridge Bay, I discovered how different things were up there. Even the RCMP could be a law unto themselves. One corporal, who had a considerable affection for the bottle, decided to shoot untied dogs. He did this right in the village from his pickup. Some of us felt this was a little dangerous and I took pictures of him doing it. A Village Council meeting was called and the issue was raised. The Village Council chairman was a drinking associate of his, but there was sufficient outcry against the RCMP that he was publicly chastised.

He took his revenge some two years later by shooting both my dogs when I was out of town. I complained to the Commissioner of the Northwest Territories and the corporal was transferred; that was my only satisfaction.

The nursing station was established in Cambridge Bay in 1956. Kay Dier, then a nurse at the Charles Camsell Hospital in Edmonton, volunteered to be the pioneer. At that time there were 120 Inuit and twelve non-natives. At the Dewline there were many labourers, but it was off-limits to natives. The contrast between the adventurous pioneer days and the more complex sociological conditions of the seventies was marked and I felt I had missed the best times in the north. Alcohol was not quite such a disaster then, and the problems brought about by increased political awareness had not arisen.

From 1956 on, we have been dealing with a marginal society and a more rapid transition, due to greater contact with the south. Kay Dier herself, in an article in 1984 in the 'Canadian Nurse', related that she was glad to have experienced the old Arctic and that the years since then had been tragic. Old friends of hers were now pathetic alcoholics.

Doctors have been resident in Cambridge Bay since 1965, most staying not more than six months. For a doctor it was not an easy place to stay, yet here I was, by some strange intersection of lines of history, in a place which fascinated me. Perhaps up here I could study more of my favourite philosopher, Ludwig Wittgenstein. First I would have to learn about this intriguing new culture and the Inuit.

Chapter 8

THE INUIT

When did the Inuit come to the Arctic? Probably they came later than the Indians came to the south. Remnants of archaeological campsites found in the 'Barren Grounds', between the Mackenzie and Hudson Bay, are those belonging to Plains Indians. Perhaps about 2000 B.C. Inuit first came to the area, according to Robert McGhee, of the National Museum in Ottawa. He did extensive archaeological work in the Coppermine area. The Paleoeskimos came from Siberia. They were bow and arrow hunters, an advance on the Plains Indian spear hunting culture.

The Paleoeskimos spread across the high Arctic areas until 1500 B.C., when a cooling trend forced everyone south. During this time the Inuit moved into the Barren Lands and the mainland for the first time. Around A.D. 1000 there was a warmer period, followed by a 'Little Ice Age', between 1600 and 1850. During this time the Eskimos developed the use of igloos and dog-teams. The climate had dictated most of these practices and inventions.

It was possible for the early migrants to walk across the Bering Straits. Geologically speaking, this area has only very recently been water covered. Three distinct waves of Inuit are known to us. The first was the Denbigh, also known as the Paleoeskimo. This period lasted from 2500 B.C. to 500 B.C. After that came the Dorset people who flourished until 800 A.D. Their culture, in turn, was replaced by the Thule Culture, which spread as far as Greenland. The language evolved, with considerable variation, from Siberia to Greenland.

Exploration has played a dominant role in the last two hundred years. After several thousand years of native culture, adapted to hunting and to a generally nomadic existence, things began to change rapidly. With the advent of missionaries, traders, civil servants, teachers and nurses, all the aboriginal peoples were accelerated into the technological age. With that came alcohol—followed closely by venereal disease and also tuberculosis, which caused many to be sent away to southern treatment centres, permanently disrupting their lives. In addition, measles, small pox, and smoking all had their effect.

Trapping was also a foreign way of life. In older times animal skins had been used only for practical purposes. Trapping, as a business, started the process of dependency on Hudson's Bay posts and on consumerism. The more the natives mixed with whites, the more they became prey to various diseases to which they possessed little immunity. These diseases caused terrible epidemics, influenza being one of the worst.

In the sixties, a measles epidemic resulted in the deaths of between 30% and 50% of the Pelly Bay children. The Canadian Government then decided that the Inuit should all live in fixed villages and in package built houses. Initially numbers were given to the Inuit, to be used instead of names. This was largely because Government officials could not pronounce the natives' names. This practice was maintained for a long time in the post-war era.

In the north there is a repeated phenomenon of instant Arctic Experts; teachers, doctors, nurses, civil servants, even tourists who are only up there for a few days. All are instant experts. Some stay one or two years and then are gone from the north for ever. I did not do much better, though I did put in the two years that Otto Schaefer hoped for, and then another couple of years here and there in the Arctic. We are just passing episodes in the lives of the locals, who see all types of 'Kabloonaks' coming and going.

Moving the Inuit into houses was a major contributing factor to the terrible tuberculosis epidemic of the fifties and sixties, which filled the Camsell Hospital and other southern centres, until treatment became easier and surveillance better. In the igloo there was a natural protection offered against the spread of the bacteria. Dr. Otto Schaefer shared with me his theory on this. When permanent housing was offered to the Inuit, naturally they took it. After all this was free housing! However, the TB bacillus also preferred the warmth of the house, and spread far more quickly, giving rise to the epidemic.

Tuberculosis prevention became a major part of the Northern Health initiative. Surveys were done with primitive equipment, rugged enough to stand travel and cold temperatures. At Bay Chimo, X-ray machines and tents were set up and everyone checked.

Patients with tuberculosis were often sent 'out' for long periods of time. To send Inuit patients out was hard. I remember one young girl who was going out for her first delivery, for medical reasons. She had to go to the Camsell Hospital in Edmonton. This meant leaving a few weeks ahead of the expected date of delivery. She lived in Spence Bay. I saw her at Cambridge Bay—all her belongings clutched in one small paper bag and tears rolling down her face.

"What is bothering you?" I asked her in the plane, on the way from her community to Cambridge Bay.

"Nothing," she answered.

"Is it your first time in a plane?" Her eyebrows went up in the characteristic "yes."

"First time to Cambridge Bay?" The eyebrows went up again.

Finally I found out that she had never been out of her community. Even to go to Cambridge Bay was stressful for her. There were 900 people and drinking and many other fearful things about which her community had warned her.

Once Inuit patients got to Edmonton it was never that bad and the young ones came back quite 'worldly'. They were looked after in Edmonton with great compassion. I remember well one Mrs. Post, who made a tremendous effort to make the Inuit patients feel at home and had been doing it for a long time.

I began to see the Inuit as neophyte villagers as well as noble hunters. To see the Eskimo as the primitive noble hunter, and to bemoan the passing of the associated era, is merely another form of colonialism. The Inuit have lost their innocence. The idyllic happiness that we perceive in their historical lifestyle, was largely the invention of anthropologists. Real life was often a desperate struggle for survival, as illustrated by the later story of a grandmother from Pelly Bay who was forced, by terrible circumstances, to let her own child die. New cultures arise by the mixing of different behaviours and manners of survival. The Inuit struck me as having a positive attitude to unknown challenges.

The Eskimo has had to adapt to the twentieth century. He cannot survive as hunter only; now he must become politician and civil servant because power and economic control have become critical issues. The sociological adaptation of the Inuit is taking place faster than ever, in the late nineties.

Certain aspects of social and environmental responsibility are harder to learn. What happened, in 1975, to the barren ground caribou illustrates this. That year the main herd ended up wintering at the village of Coppermine. Sixty thousand caribou remained within several miles of the village. Whenever I came in with Tug, the pilot, we had to buzz the runway to clear the caribou away. Unfortunately laws in Canada do not apply to all equally. While there can be cultural interpretation, hunting laws are for the preservation of species and should be enforced nation wide. Such was not the case that winter. Close to 2000 caribou were slaughtered indiscriminately by the Inuit and few of the animals were eaten. Many carcasses littered the surrounding country and the airport. In spring the carcasses were bulldozed into the sea.

I went on one long hunting trip with some Eskimo friends and once again experienced a lack of responsibility in hunting. Travelling 80 to 100 miles south from Cambridge Bay, we found a herd of thirty-five caribou. We were in the area of Buchan Hills, north of Bay Chimo. It was a beautiful day; the sun was shining and we were warm. The rolling hills were a contrast to Cambridge Bay and the scene was surrealistic; all white with nothing to disturb it except the animals.

We spotted the herd of caribou as we came over the brow of a hill on our snowmobiles. There was no escape for them. We got them from the side, as they ran along a narrow valley. The first seven were shot, the others just wounded. It mattered not, for they could not run far and we tracked them all down, until every last one went down.

The poor animals limped along, on shattered legs, until they were put out of their misery. I felt that some of this was for my benefit. In the village my friend Allan was more subdued, but out here I was on his terms. This was his natural country; I was the intruder. I like to think he was not always that cruel to the animals and that he did it just to show me that this was his land, out here away from the town.

The final killing involved slow teasing which was plain cruelty. I have never enjoyed hunting, other than some smaller game, since that day. Jack Hornby reports in his diary, from his Barrenland trips, in 1923, the same blatant cruelty. Such cruelty may be an expression of the Inuit's own indifference to pain. Any concern—and I did show some—was seen as a weakness.

On the way back my snowmobile seized up. I was towing one passenger and twelve caribou, on a sled. We left it all, cached the caribou and Allan and I went over, on his machine, to Hope Bay Silver Mines. Peter Avaluk was living there with his family and we wanted to make sure the skidoo would be safe. Arriving there after several hours of snowmobiling, we were just in time for cooked baby seal liver. After that, we consumed homebrew and left at 2 a.m., feeling no pain! This was a good thing because Peter promptly fell off his machine. I was sitting on the sled, being towed by his snowmobile and he came right under the runners beneath me. The sleds are twenty feet long, with steel runners. I feared that he would not get up at all. I think he broke a rib, but he did not complain and we carried on.

We travelled at full bore, not an easy task in hilly country with a twenty foot, wood and steel sled. To go down a fairly steep hill meant never letting the sled catch up. We arrived back at camp at breakfast time.

To be out travelling or hunting with the Inuit is to partake in one of life's great pleasures. They are happy and relaxed and do not feel constrained by the artificiality of the community. I was now out in their natural environment, as opposed to the towns, and they felt honoured to share it with me. There was a sense of freedom and exhilaration which was rarely felt.

Exhibiting self-reliance is important in order to gain respect from the Inuit. On my return trip to fetch my skidoo, I was sent back with Allan's father. I think he had specific instructions to make sure we were safe but not to help too much. John Robertson, a friend and local teacher, came along as he was one of the few whites who had done some travelling on the land. When John's snowmobile broke down, the old man walked off and left us to figure out what was wrong. Allan was trying to teach us a lesson. He often told me that the Inuit regarded whites as children in many ways. They respected and feared our knowledge and technology, yet felt superior to us in learning to be 'real men.' It was definitely a male thing, but the women had to be tough as well.

If you don't learn this self-reliance in the Arctic you are a danger to yourself and others. The degree of hardship one can endure varies and I had the utmost respect for most hunters. A friend of mine, Isaac, had been on a hunting trip with his brother and grandfather when their skidoo broke down. They were many miles into the interior of Victoria Island, on a polar bear hunt. Isaac and his brother left their grandfather by the sled, with a caribou which they had shot. He would be fine for several days with that. Later, when I checked Isaac over for exposure he told me the tale:

"My brother and I walked and walked and walked. After three days he argued with me over the direction and went another way. I walked on for some days without sleeping. On the last day I lay down to sleep but was woken by the sound of a swan flying over me. I got up and made it into the village."

Isaac's brother, who worked as a civil servant, may have lost some of his survival skills. He was convinced the direction they were walking in was wrong, and took off on his own. Isaac's grandfather got bored waiting and hiked in, covering the distance in four days. Isaac had walked for six.

Bobby, Isaac's brother, was never seen again. We searched for his body again in the spring, but to no avail.

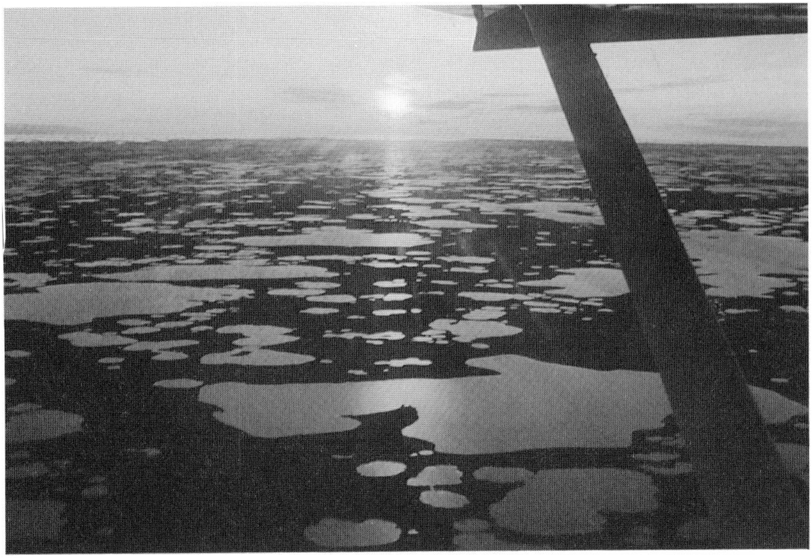

"I gaze at the flat, flat ground beneath me ..."

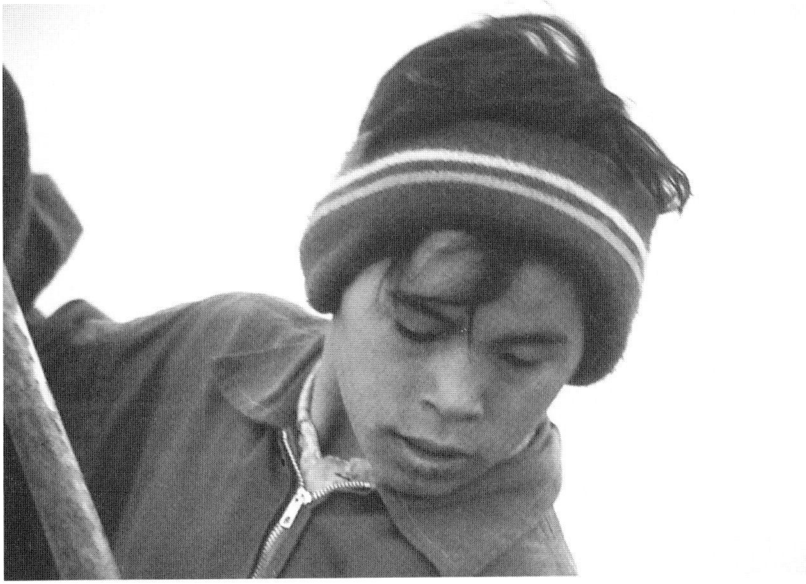

"I became good friends with the Hakungak family, George, who is just a teenager ..."

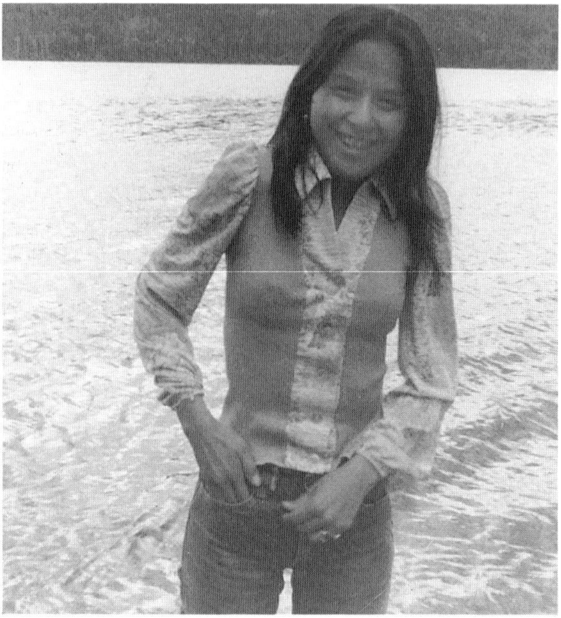

"Rosie, who was about 12 or 13 at the time, was the oldest ..."

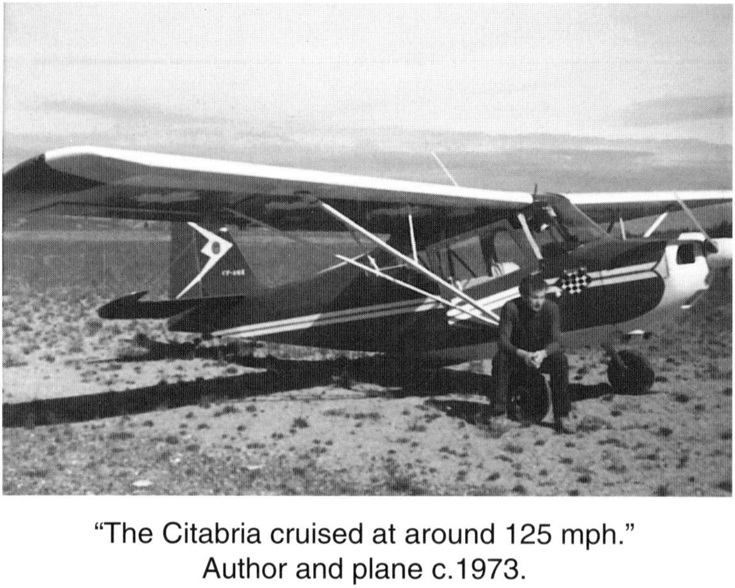

"The Citabria cruised at around 125 mph."
Author and plane c.1973.

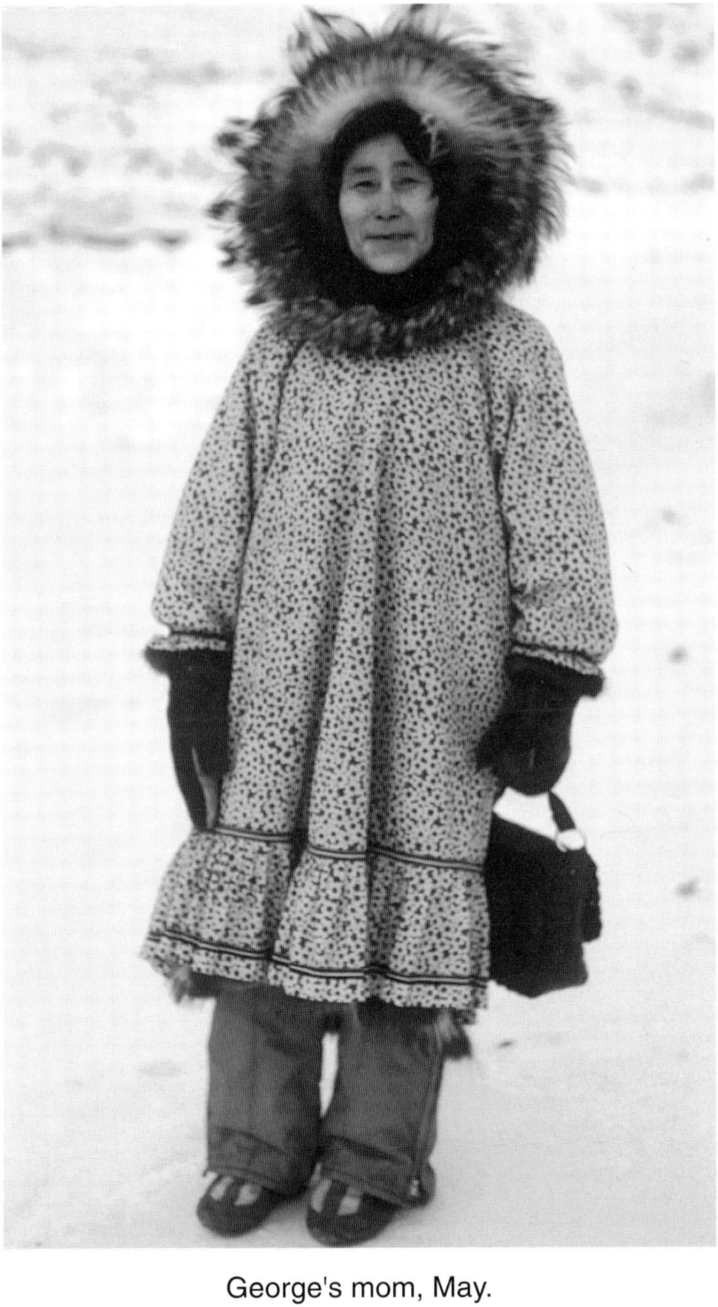

George's mom, May.

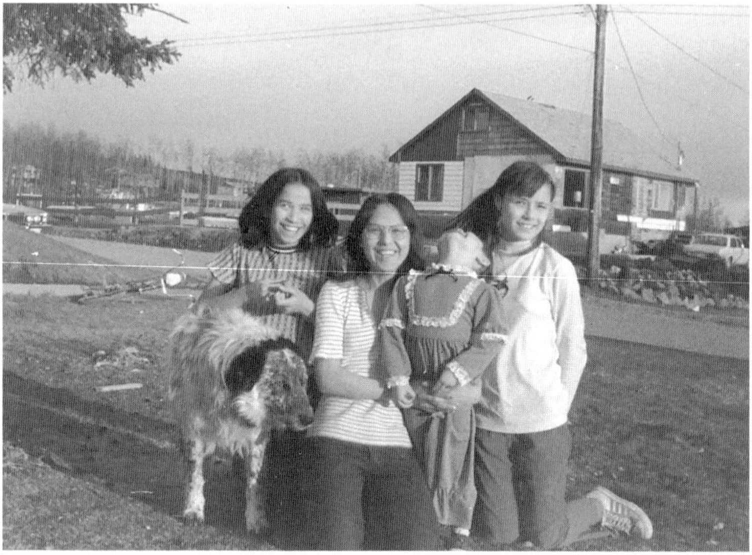

Ruffy the dog, Sylvia,(a friend) Rosie, Sabrina
and Corrina, 1976.

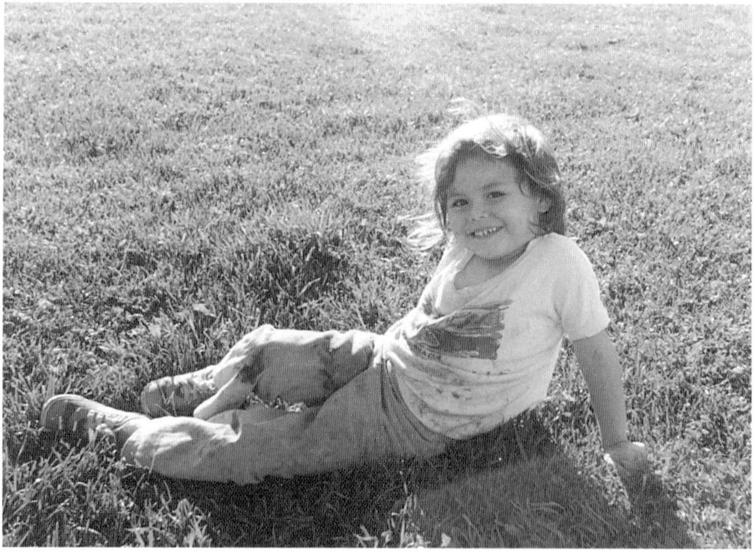

Sabrina.

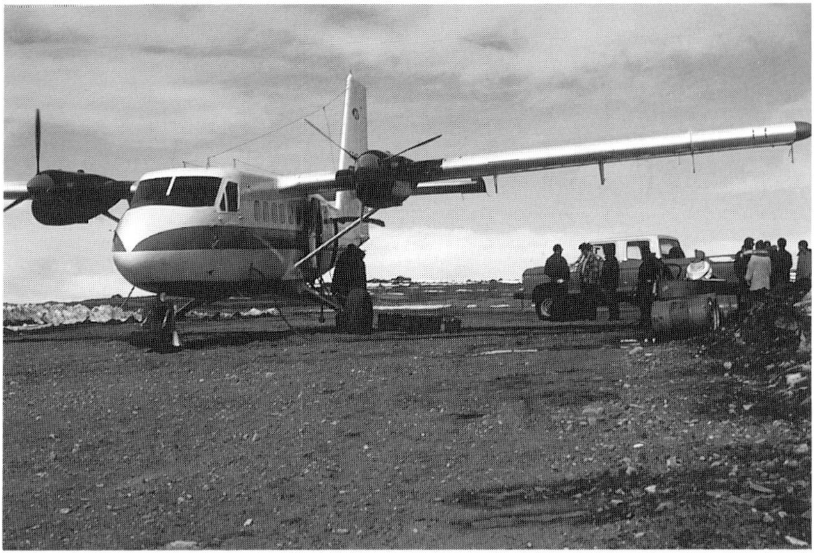

"We were flown up to Cambridge Bay in a De Havilland Twin Otter–luggage, dogs, the lot."

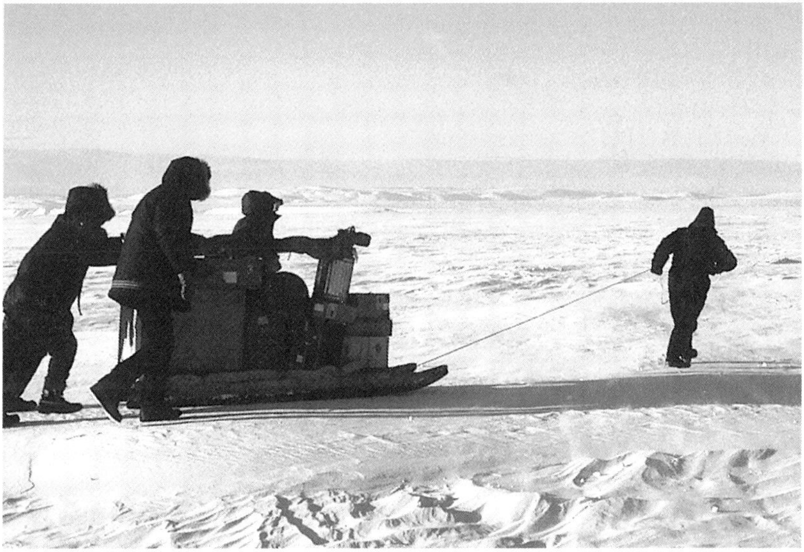

" At Bay Chimo X-ray machines and tents were set up..."

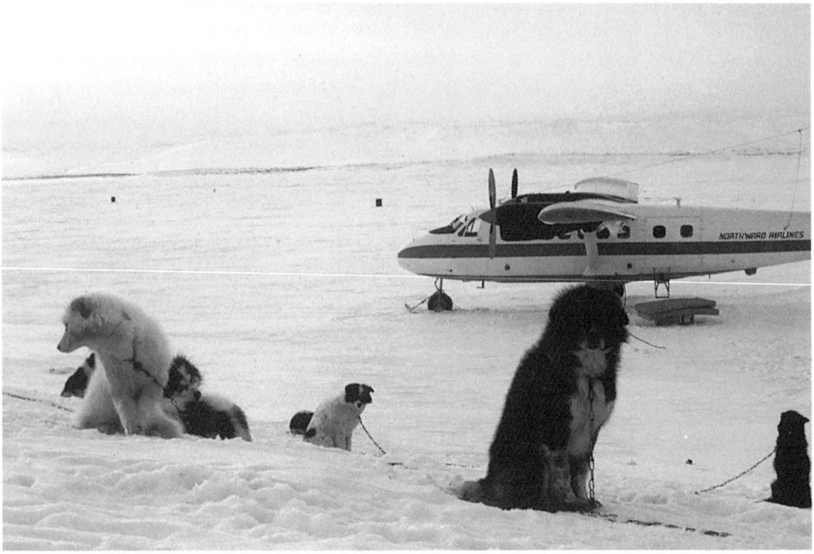

"We landed on the sea ice on wheels, in a foot of snow."

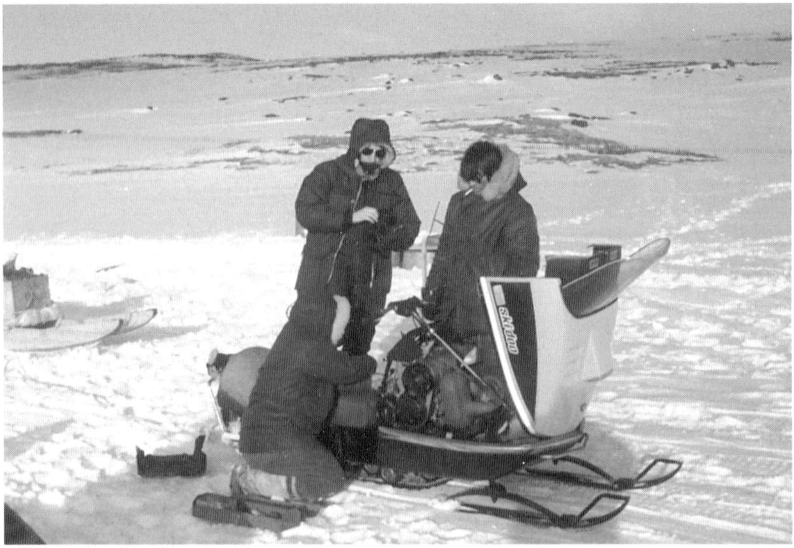

"We stop after five minutes of travel over frozen sea..."

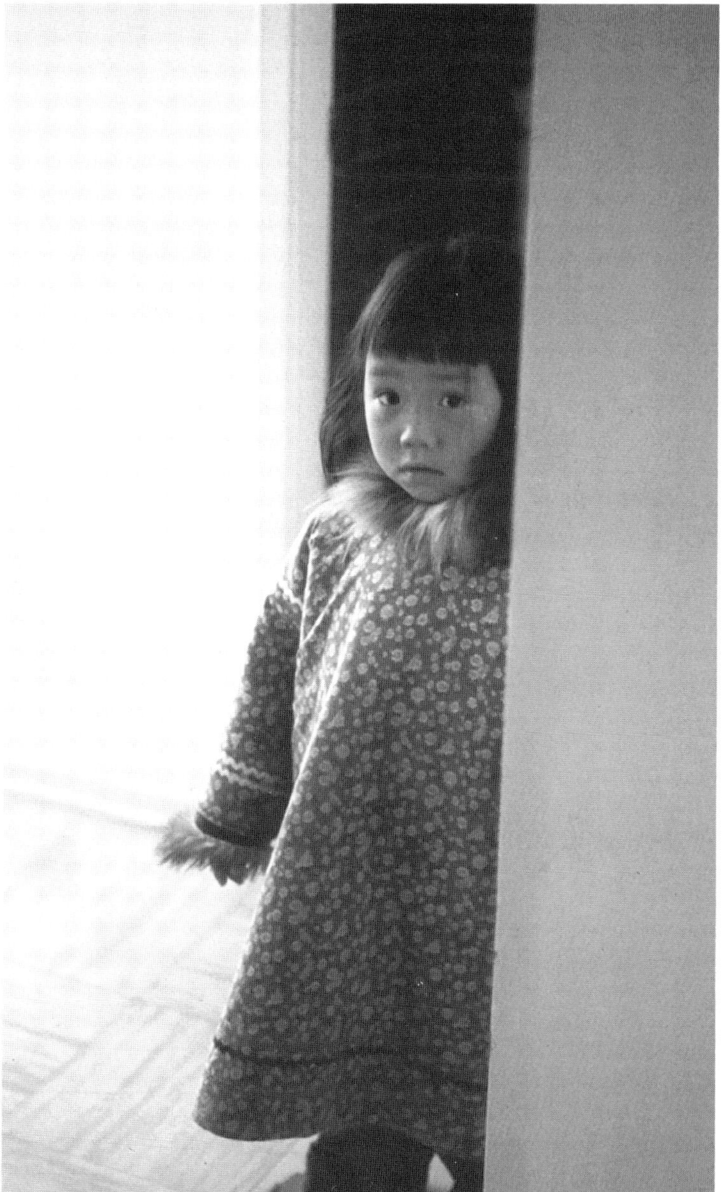

"At the end of the clinic I would see a little child standing by the door."

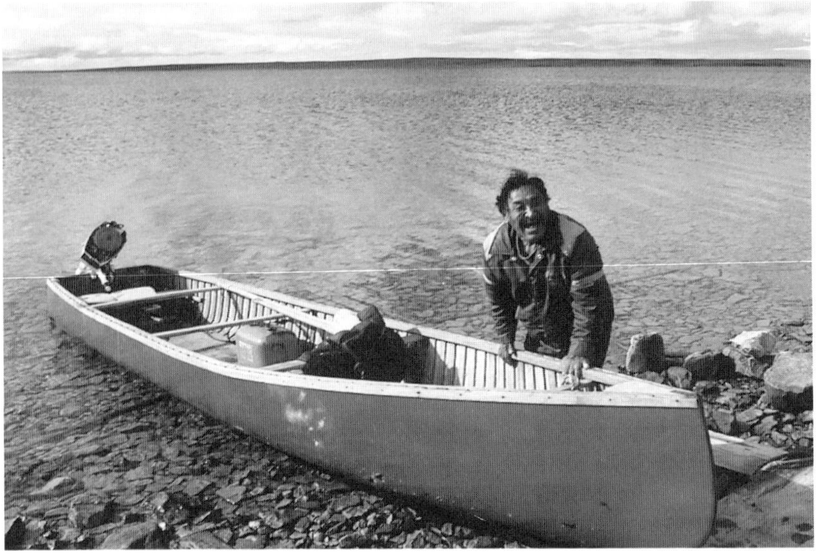

"Mahik became like a grandfather,although speaking about as much English as I did Inuktitut."

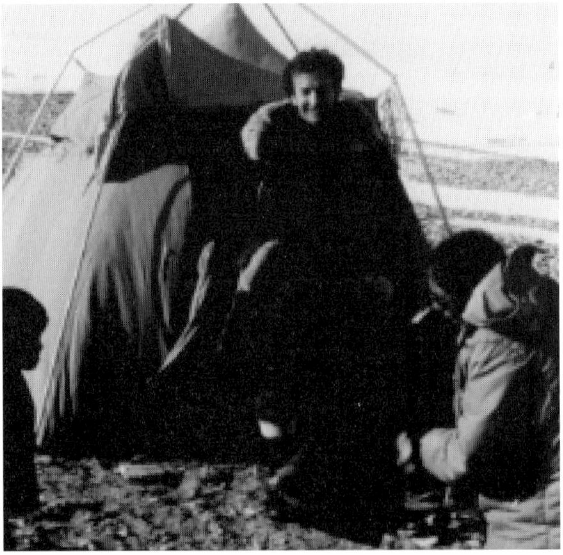

"House calls were undertaken ... this was at times to a tent in the middle of nowhere..."

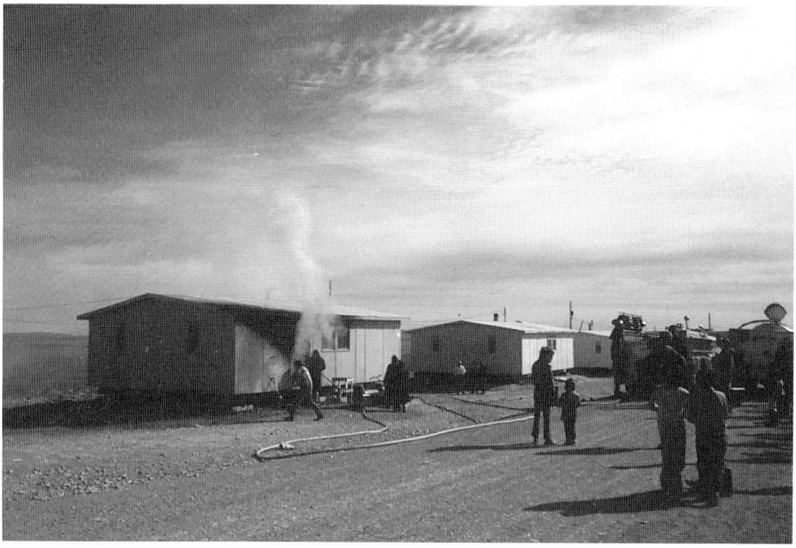

"Someone had passed out with a cigarette still burning ... the result was four dead."

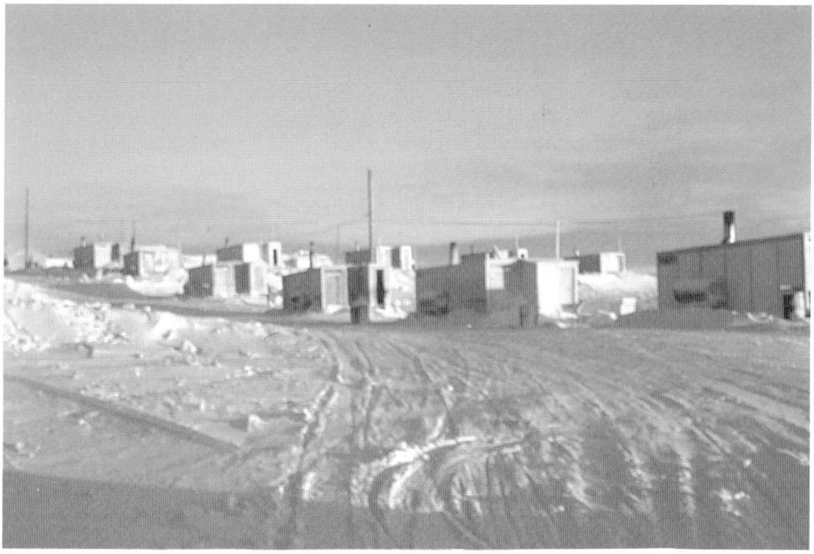

"...built as a temporary housing measure some ten years earlier..."

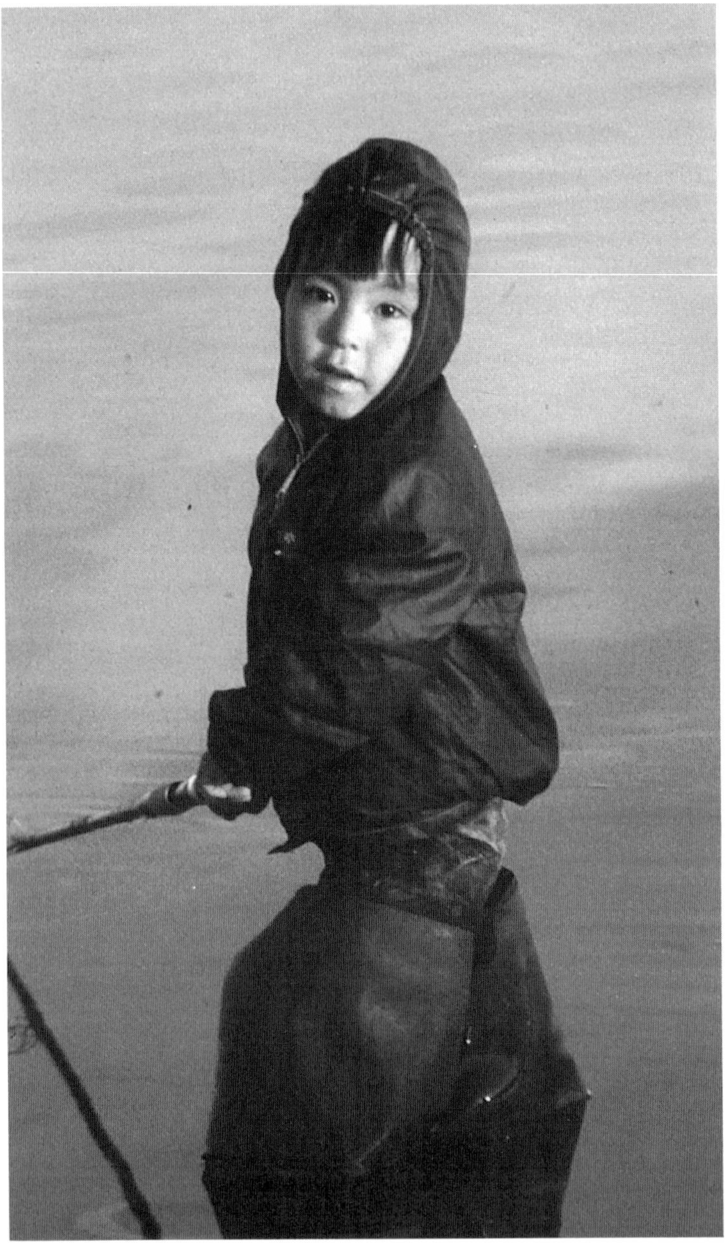

" The sun is beaming down, out of a cloudless sky, though it is 2 a.m."

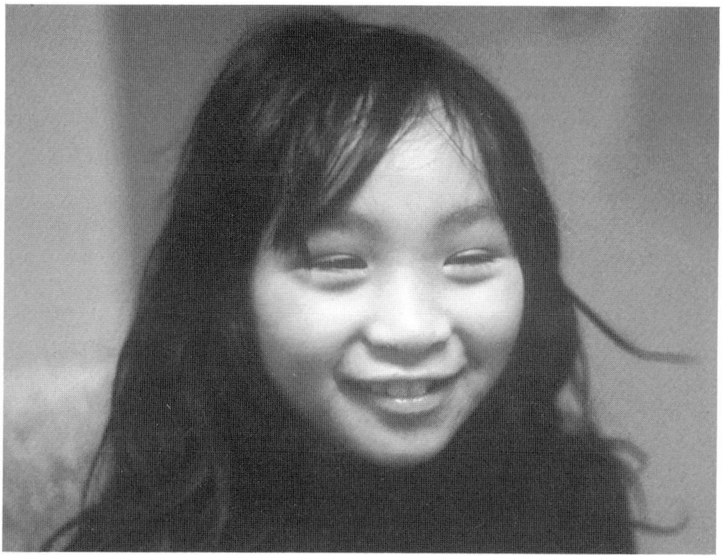

"...we were met by the Nakasook and Kamoayok children." Vera Kamoayuk. 1975.

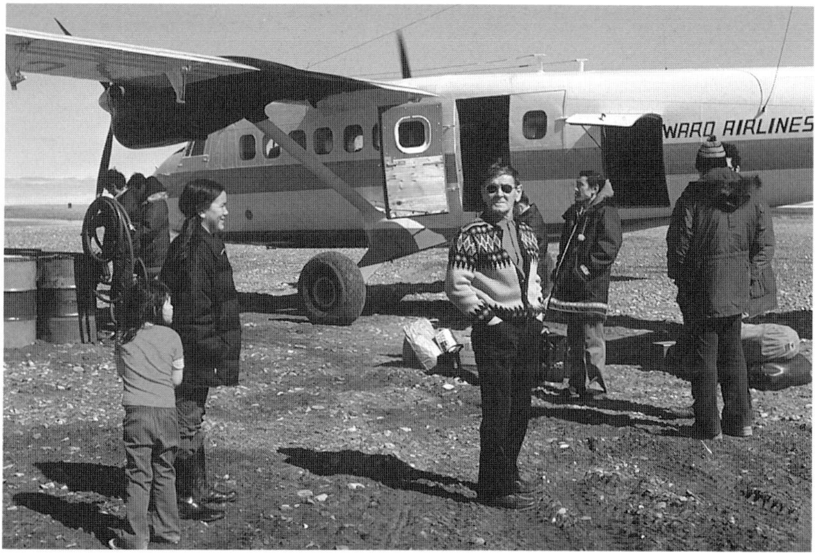

Ernie Lyall and family. 1975.

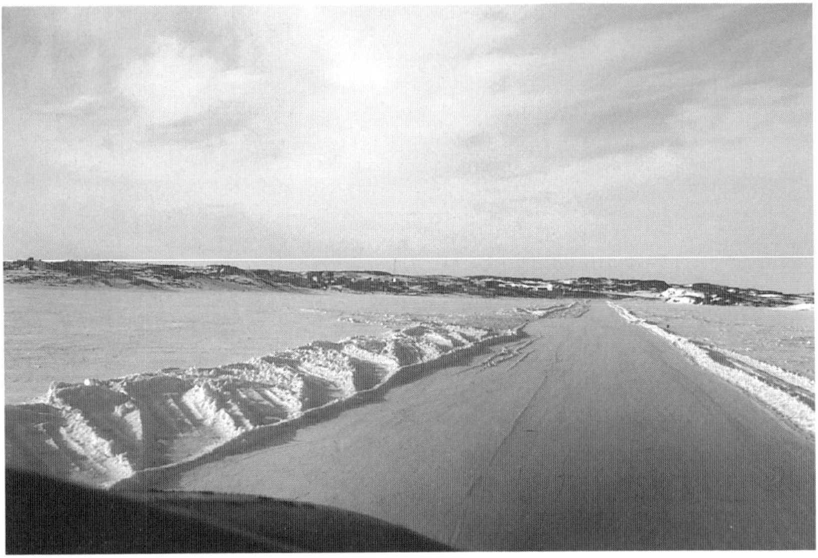

"In the winter we would land on the sea ice."

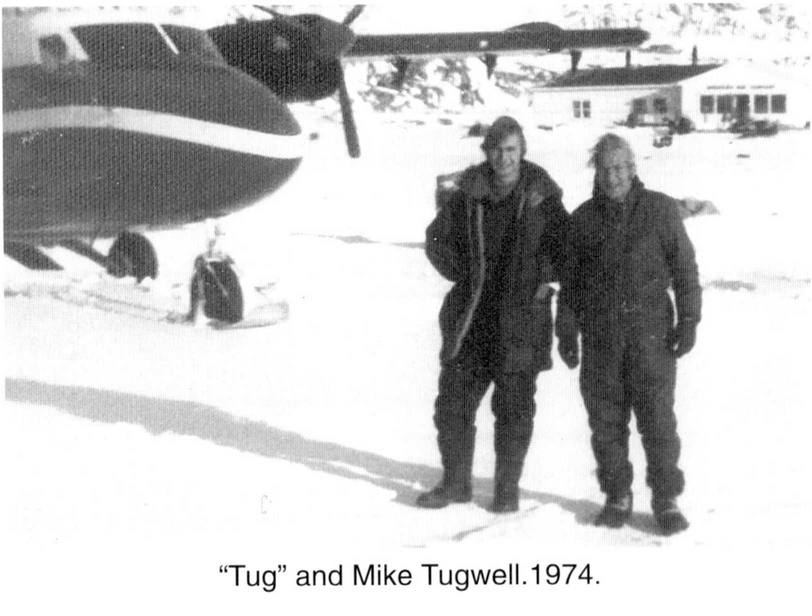

"Tug" and Mike Tugwell.1974.

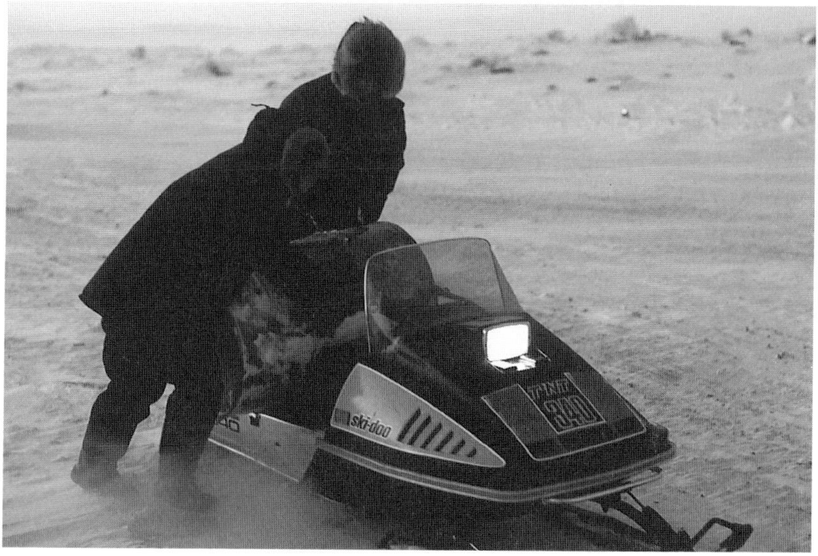

"Fuelling up from barrels at -35°F in a wind is a good learning experience for anyone."

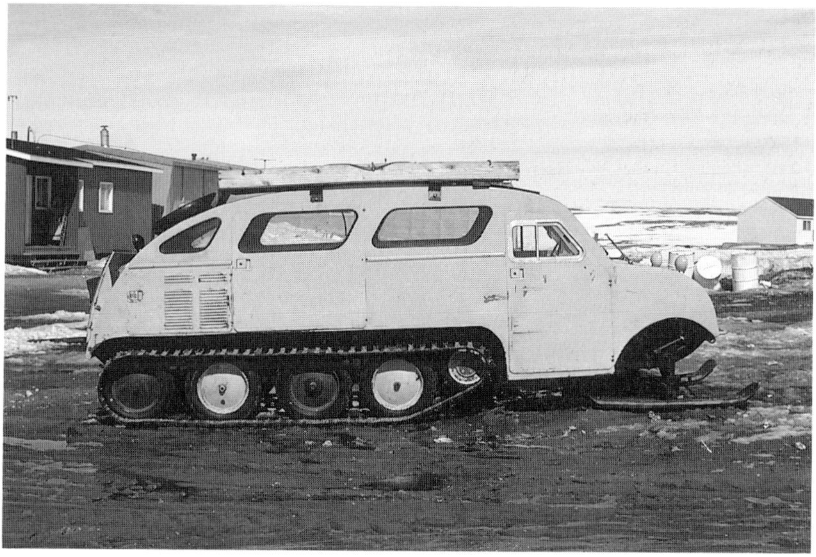

"The Nodwell is an enclosed snow machine..."

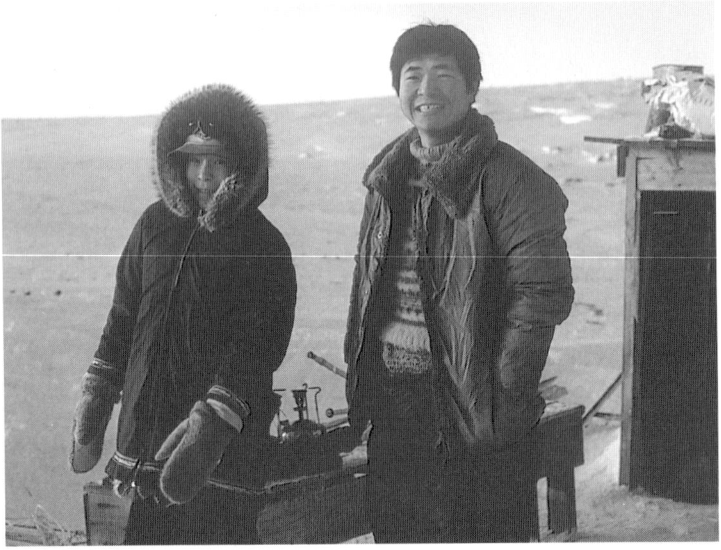

"Even George was complaining of the cold..."
Naomi Uemura and George Hakungak

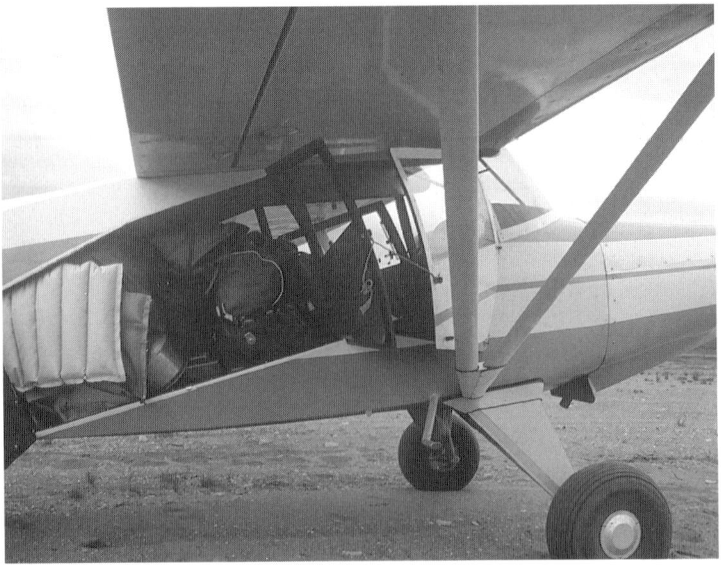

The Maule M5-235 loaded for Arctic flying

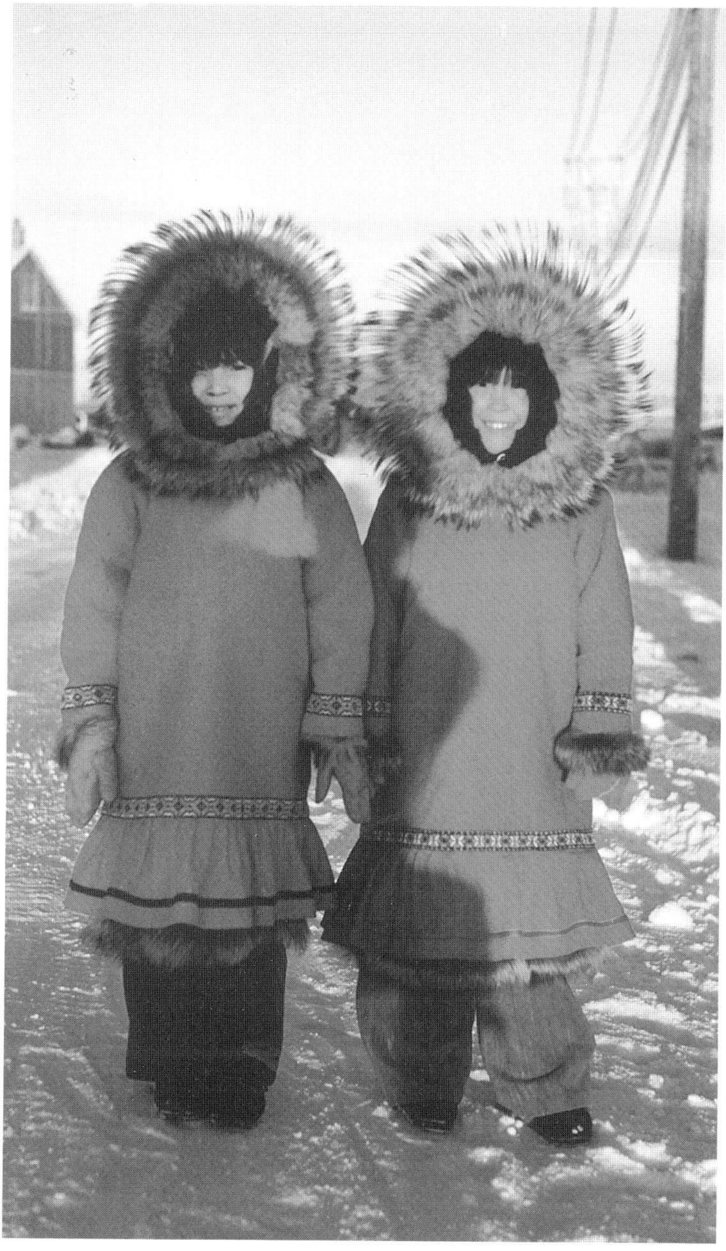

Two young Inuk girls, Cambridge Bay.

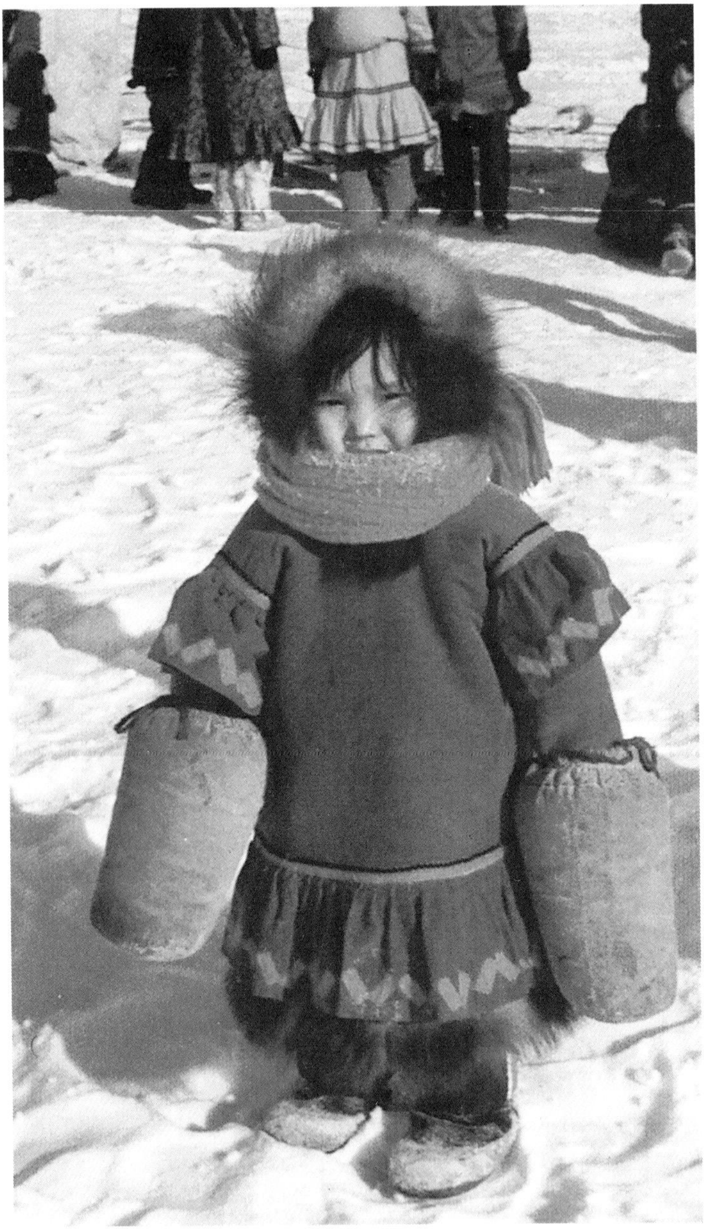

Jennifer, Cambridge Bay.

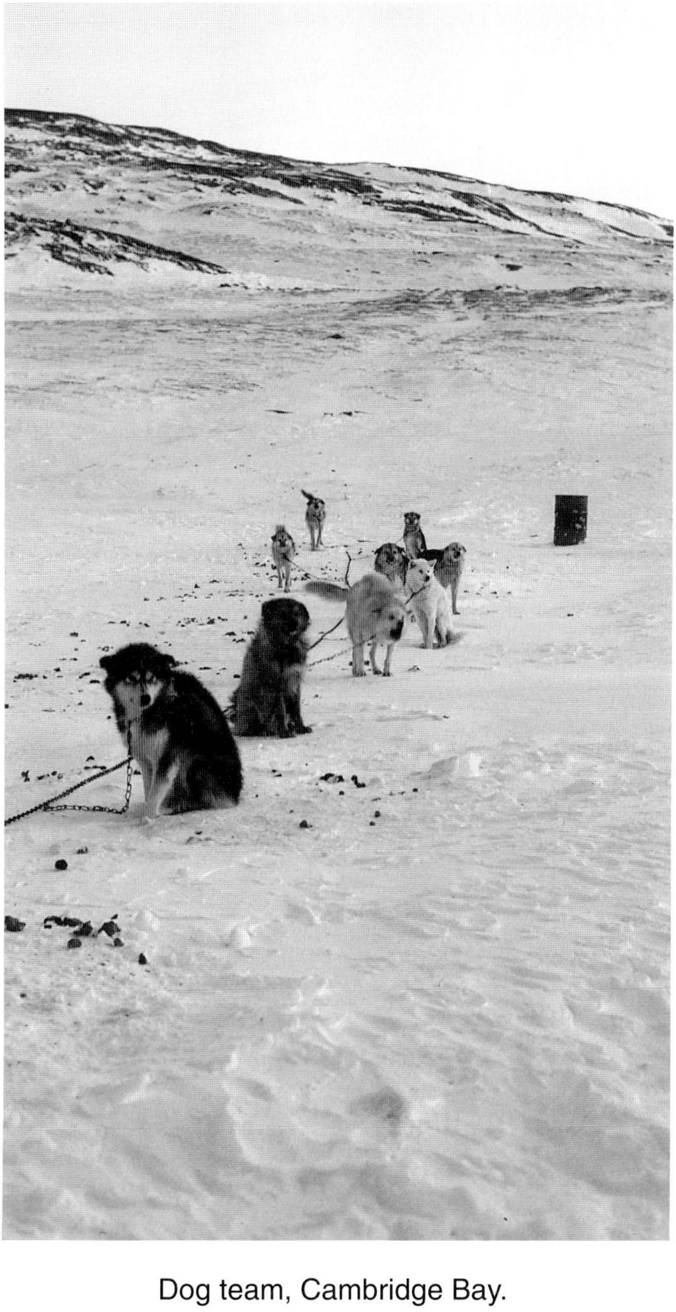

Dog team, Cambridge Bay.

Chapter 9

ARCTIC MEDICINE, ARCTIC FLYING AND A SNOWMOBILE TRIP

In April 1974, 'Tug' Tugwell, the Northward Airlines local chief pilot, flew me down to Bay Chimo in the Twin Otter. We landed on the sea ice on wheels, in a foot of snow. I was expecting to see skis on all three wheels but the Twin Otter has a nosewheel ski only for the Arctic. There is not enough snow in the Arctic to warrant more! We loaded in a young Eskimo boy who had a dislocated hip, and Tug made a short take-off. The flight was just over one hour. Back at Cambridge Bay we were able to get an X-Ray done, confirm the diagnosis and then try to do something about the problem. Hips can be hard to reduce, but with IV valium I was able to get the boy relaxed enough that his hip popped back in, with a small manipulation.

A week later we were back down to Bay Chimo for a flu epidemic, probably started by us the previous week, and I saw six cases of pneumonia out of a population of forty. I decided to bring out the worst cases. One little baby had already died and was 'buried' in an old blanket on top of a little hill. As there was not even radio contact here, I gave an instant outpost training course to Jessie Hakungak. One other patient, an old man, had also died during the week and was outside wrapped in a caribou hide. His grandchildren took me up to see the body as I was still supposed to pronounce him dead. There could be little doubt in this case and the animals had already begun to fulfill their role in nature. The children were unperturbed by this.

In Cambridge Bay we did bury in coffins, but the coffins stayed on top of the ground until sometime in summer, when a machine could dig. Children would occasionally wander into the nursing station bringing parts of a body with them.

On the return trip from Bay Chimo, I started to learn how to fly the Twin Otter CF-QUB, but Tug took over for the landing as ice-fog had now formed and we were almost in a white-out.

The landing involved a careful approach on the VOR, the VHF Omni Range, even to below minimums on some medevacs. A cross position was kept using the ADF, or Automatic Direction Finder, and there were two of these at Cambridge Bay. The VOR was new and was a luxury; Tug had landed many times in the past with only the ADFs. I developed a great admiration for these northern pilots. Many a time a nurse or doctor was helped out of a desperate situation by a pilot willing to attempt a flight in unpleasant conditions. Often, when all routine flying was cancelled, we would find Tug, and other pilots, still willing to go on a medevac. To my mind they were the unsung heroes of the north and were a lifeline to us.

The pilots cannot make medical decisions but having a doctor with a pilot's license seemed to be helpful. I went north partly to fly, and felt that I should gain as much experience as I could. I wanted to be able to weigh the balance of risks. Various factors would be involved in medevac decisions, including weather, safety of pilot and crew, and the cost of the flight against the degree of medical urgency.

At times, a doctor would have to turn down a request for a plane, as there might be an element of panic, on the part of the nurse, out of proportion to the state of the patient. Yet again, as happened to me on one occasion, it might be evident that the patient was going to die anyway and there really was not much advantage to having him or her die enroute, unless there was a chance for helpful intervention. These were difficult and emotional decisions, but I had to be firm that I was not risking pilots and other medical personnel, for a hopeless case. My knowledge as a pilot enabled me to talk, both to nurses and pilots, with a degree of confidence, and to weigh the issues.

MAY 1ST 1974: *Sometimes I think I am just here to fill a post. I fill in long days and nights doing nothing. Am I getting 'bushed' already? I've only been here a month! Today it is -25°F and blowing a storm. It gets dusky for only two hours around midnight. Cardboard over the windows does not seem to help. We stayed up all night, then slept at midday for two hours. Our friends are important; Tugwells, Robertsons, and the occasional visit to the strange world of the Dewline station.*

Later in May I went to Coppermine, 350 miles to the west, to visit Martha and 'Tops'. These two nurses put in many years of northern service. They would babble away and complain about everything and everyone, yet they loved their community and put their hearts and souls into the job. I enjoyed every visit there. Tops died some years later, hiking on Baffin Island, when her heavy backpack caused her to lose her footing, while crossing a river. Martha and 'Tops' had been together for twenty years, working in Northern Ontario and then the Arctic. 'Tops' was originally from Holland and I believe Martha was from eastern Canada.

Next I went over to Holman Island to visit one of the most isolated nurses, Pam Boyd. Pam was one of those highly trained nurses with obstetrical experience, who could be safely placed in a community where many modern doctors would fear to stay, lest their inadequacy show. In settlements like this, people want to meet you and know you, so you are not just a voice on the erratic HF radio. To establish a working rapport with an excellent nurse like Pam, one had to interpret the unsaid things on the radio. If she told me she wanted a plane, I never questioned it.

A good example of the stupidity of bureaucracy descended on poor Pam. She had severely sprained, or maybe broken, her ankle on one occasion. She was unable to get me on the radio, so had given herself a shot of demerol. I was not able to get in there for two weeks and she was doing OK by then, but her administrative boss had made life hell for her because one vial of demerol had been used on a 'non-patient'. These were isolation pressures which made my blood boil.

When the plane landed at Holman it was welcomed by everyone. It is hard not to welcome a plane which lands on your one main street! The planes usually made a preliminary pass to clear children and dogs out of the way. Even the DC-3 would land right there. Holman was such a lovely settlement; I would have been happy to live there and not in Cambridge Bay. I went as often as I could to do clinics and generally stayed for a day or two.

MAY 14TH, 1974: *Whilst in Holman this time, Pam took me to visit the artist Kalvak, and also Eliazbeth Banksland, the daughter of Natkusiak. This was especially thrilling to me. Natkusiak (Billy Banksland) had accompanied Stefansson on his travels off the sea ice around here during the First World War. I went for an ice-fishing trip with Alec Banksland and his wife Elizabeth and was infected by their merriment and sense of humour. Kalvak was a famous artist but also an infamous shaman. I had to honour her and follow the wise advice of Pam as to how to behave suitably. Before I leave Holman, on each visit, I have to go to her house, take her blood pressure and inject her somewhere with sterile water. She does not know what is in the syringe but it is some part of my shamanistic belongings which she does not have!*

She is reputed to be capable of turning into a polar bear and of putting hexes on people. I certainly do not want her to get upset with me!

According to Elizabeth Banksland, Kalvak had supposedly caused a person to die by casting a spell. Kalvak had a fertile artistic imagination and Fr. Metayer had made a collection of tapes with her. These were interviews between himself and Kalvak, in Inuktitut, in which she described some of the symbolism in her art work.

MAY 15TH, 1974: *In QBV on the way home....... We are suspended in a timeless zone up here at 9000'; the sun barely set. There is a red glow over the distant clouds. I sit in the second row, just ahead of the prop blades. Sometimes I look out at these props and listen to the ice thudding into the side of the fuselage. I think it would take my kneecaps, if the ice came through the plane. I am in a state of deep awe towards nature. Up front, the two pilots, Tug and Ken Murphy, sit flying for the ninth hour today. The control panel glows a comforting red. They light up cigarettes to keep themselves company. 1500 miles flying today and some of that quite unusual instrument flying.*

My mind goes to Antoine de Sainte-Exupéry's description of the early Andes pilots. To get in to Holman they have to let down over the beacon at Holman, usually 'in the soup', then go past the cliffs at 2000' outbound, then let down over the sea to 500' and edge back in to catch a glimpse of the main street. No DME, no glide slope. All eyes and instincts; every approach a calculated risk.

MAY 16TH, 1974: *Down to Yellowknife with a two year old with bronchiolitis and back via Bay Chimo, where all is now settled. Jessie had gone ahead, using my primitive criteria, and put several people on antibiotics. Back in to Cambridge with 200' ceiling. Nine hours flying today.*

MAY 18TH, 1974: *Visit to Pelly Bay, 500 miles east, brief clinic, then Hugh Stephenson from Cambridge Bay Government office asks me if I'd like to join him and two Inuit on a snowmobile trip to Gjoa Haven. This will be a twenty hour skidoo ride across the Boothia Peninsula. Wow! Right through the area where James Ross first mapped the Magnetic North Pole and where Simpson explored. Possibly very few whites have been here since Rasmussen's trip in the twenties. Too good a chance to miss, though I am inadequately clothed.*

We go with two snowmobiles and 'komatiks', sleds with steel runners, not like the old mud-glazed ones used with dog teams. The food is frozen raw caribou; a first for me, so I quickly buy one can of tomato soup to take along. Emiliano Kringorn and his cousin from Pelly Bay guide us. Communications are sparse but Hugh has a little Inuktitut. I travel behind Emiliano, on his komatik; he glances at my attire as we leave and says nothing.

We stop after five minutes of travel over frozen sea and check spark plugs etc. This is the pre-flight check! Then off at full throttle and back-jarring speed across thirty miles of sea to reach the Boothia Peninsula. I am excited and already freezing! According to my reading, we are following Knud Rasmussen's route on the Fifth Thule Expedition, in the twenties. He went with dog teams. We go up Simpson Lake and then skidoo along the Murchison River.

By the time we get to the Murchison I am really freezing, but say nothing. We put on extra socks and Hugh gets a caribou parka from his guide. I am already picturing the one I will have made as soon as I get to Cambridge Bay. I sing loudly to counteract the cold and stop my ribs from shivering uncontrollably. Finally we make camp and have tea and heat up some hairy caribou soup. I am in heaven after about one hour in the sleeping bag!

The next day we continue across the open sea of the Rasmussen Basin, nearby the spot where, just 130 years ago, Franklin and his men were doomed by not knowing that they could get through this very passage. We cross Rae Straits and see some seals, and also the very mirages that Ross must have seen. It becomes a white-out after a while, but now I am adapting better to the cold.

Once the distraction of the cold is overcome, I become aware of the tremendous beauty all around me. Yet what is there around me? Open spaces, silence, total whiteness, and yet a mystical sense of unreality, coupled with a feeling that I am an extremely lucky human being, just to be here. I am again, as so many times in the Arctic, face to face with myself. The worst thing that might happen is that I might die; and that is not so bad.

I sit on the back of the twenty-foot sled, bouncing over every ice ridge, travelling at 30 mph. I am inhaling fair quantities of ice and snow from the snowmobile, and loving it! I am quite happy that someone knows in what direction to travel, however, as everything looks the same to me.

By evening we are in Gjoa Haven, on King William Island. As we snowmobile into the harbour, I am so excited. Now I will get to see the harbour and village where Amundsen wintered over on his successful journey through the N.W. Passage, in 1903-1905. It is flat and desolate but to me it looks beautiful.

We arrive in the middle of a party. Willy Laserich, an old Arctic pilot, is there, as is Gaby Gelee an artist and sculptor. We discuss long into the light evening, the psychology of colour and the origins of language. There is no sense of time or rush. I never see Gaby again, but remember that discussion to this day. There is so much time for a quiet glass of Glenfiddich in the late evening, but unfortunately we only have beer! Willy Laserich has already been up here for many years and is something of a living legend. He knows most of the people in the area by their first names, and has earned much respect in the north. Willy flies mostly his Single Otter or his newer acquisition, the DC-6. Talking to him, I have the feeling that if I ever need a plane, he will be right there.

Chapter 10

UNUSUAL MEDICAL PROBLEMS IN THE NORTH

The Inuit are stoic, and I had first hand evidence of their high pain thresholds when my friend Alan dislocated his patella, on crashing his skidoo on an ice-fishing trip. I popped it back in, while we were out on the trail. He was limping around town for a few days but never came to see me at the clinic. He did not complain of pain throughout. Diagnosis is sometimes difficult when pain is not obvious. The little Inuit children would wander into the nursing station but would not say that they had come to see the doctor. Often no parents would come with them. At the end of the clinic I would see a little child standing by the door.

"Have you come to see me?" I would enquire.

This would be answered by a quick raise of the eyebrows. This is the easy way of saying "yes" but one has to be quick to spot it. Then I would say:

"Are you sick?"

This would turn out to be the wrong question and could be met with eyebrows up, or a really fast wrinkling of the nose, meaning "No." By now I would be thinking ahead, throwing out all medical school training and going to direct questioning:

"Are your ears infected?"

If this drew a nose wrinkle then I'd go to bellyache or throat questions. System by system would follow until the eyebrows went up. They did not teach me this in medical school!

Young children might wander into the nursing station and complain of a 'belly-ache' that had been present for a few days. I would find an advanced appendicitis, possibly already forming an abscess. This did not constitute an emergency. I would give them antibiotics and arrange a plane at convenience. The doctors in Yellowknife were experts at operating on late appendicitis. We had only one bowel fistula formation, a complication of late surgery, in two and a half years.

House calls were undertaken, in the settlements or the summer camps, but they sometimes involved a flying trip of a few hundred miles before the visit! This was at times to a tent in the middle of nowhere and would always be a social as well as a business occasion.

Alcohol has proven to be a big problem up north. Research has shown that Indians and Inuit may lack alcohol dehydrogenase, an enzyme that metabolizes alcohol and gets it out of the system more quickly. Without this enzyme there may be an accumulation of acetaldehyde and consequent toxic behaviour. Cambridge Bay was not 'dry' at this time and we had to line up at the Hudson's Bay store on Saturday mornings for our allotted two dozen beers. There was no other liquor available in town, so Saturday was a big drunk. With old Mahik, an Inuk in his seventies, I used to share an occasional glass of whisky. He kept a bottle locked up in a trunk under his bed. Mahik became like a grandfather to me, although speaking about as much English as I did Inuktitut.

The Inuit made a lot of homebrew or 'imiogak'. This was made with sugar, rice, beans, water and some yeast. If no yeast was readily available then bread and pilot biscuits would suffice. It could be drunk the same day it was made, though we could never figure out how it could have any alcohol by then! Shortly before I finally left Cambridge Bay, two of us were out duck hunting, far out on the sea ice, when we came across the tent of 'Shorty' Aptalok and his wife. They invited me in for a farewell drink. I sat and drank a couple of glasses of the mixture, then said that we had to depart and headed back to the mainland. I felt distinctly heady but not 'drunk'.

At drinking times, fights would erupt very quickly. Peculiar jealousies would arise and all control would be lost.

One night, when it was -45°F, there was a call for the fire brigade. At those temperatures, with a wooden house and volunteer fire brigade, it might seem a hopeless situation, yet they tried their hardest. There had been some drinking and someone had passed out with a cigarette still burning. The result was four dead and one surviving child, aged fourteen, who was not at home, at the time. Two little children were asphyxiated, as were their parents. It was a terrible tragedy, felt all the more by me because they were Mahik's family. There was no actual fire; just a flash burn of paint followed by smoke. The bodies were all charred black and were brought into the nursing station very quickly in case anybody might possibly be still alive. The stench was overbearing.

We put the bodies into body bags and placed them all in the 'morgue', which was a disused garage. Next day I received a phone call from the RCMP:

"Hey Doc, I need a blood sample from one of the bodies."

"You've got to be kidding! They've been outside at -45°F all night. We won't get blood."

"Well would you mind trying anyway?"

We headed over to the garage, as he needed carbon monoxide levels to complete the investigation. It was still miserably cold. The crackling, frozen, plastic body bags were unzipped and I poked a needle into the heart of one adult victim. Amazingly I got some blood! My hands were freezing, but the poor RCMP corporal was even colder. He had to open his jacket and shirt, then hold a cigarette lighter under the syringe as I drew blood, then immediately transfer the vial close to his chest, to prevent the sample from freezing. The specimen worked and did confirm the cause of death.

The family wanted a Pentecostal burial. I had to go and help get the bodies into the coffins. I'm not sure why I had to do that; by default I think! The body bags made a musical crinkling sound when moved at these temperatures. We, being neophytes in the burial business, had placed the bodies with the arms at the side, but without enough attention to position. The coffin lids did not fit on! We had to transport the coffins down to the church with the arms sticking out on one side, then place them in front of the altar, arms towards the preacher, coffin lids partly covering them. The ceremony was completed later that day; somewhat macabre, I thought, but we could not help it.

The cold could catch one unawares if precautions were not taken, and seemingly harmless situations would quickly become dangerous. One short fishing trip was a good example of this.

A visiting psychiatrist had expressed a desire to go ice fishing. Dr. Ken Mackay was based in Yellowknife and was up visiting Cambridge Bay with a friend, Dr. Ross Wheeler. We went as far as Grenier Lake, just three miles north of the village. It was fairly cold and when we got there we found my Inuktitut language teacher, his wife, and 48 empty cans of beer. This somewhat spoiled the idyllic ice fishing but we stayed there anyway.

An ominous wind came up, so we sent the 'drunks' ahead of us and then headed in ourselves. Sure enough a 'pirktok', or small blizzard, blew in. My skidoo broke down, leaving four of us on one snowmobile and sled. We waited by the trail for a while in increasingly blowing snow. Soon a local hunter came by, and, barely slowing down, indicated that we should hop on the sled. He had just shot a caribou. Three of us jumped quickly, but Ken only managed to grab an antler at the back of the sled. He was dragged in to town, half on the ground! It seemed to take only ten minutes to get in, but by then he was hypothermic and frost-bitten. We popped him into a warm bath at home and then, being good physicians, poured ourselves some medicinal whisky, but told Ken he'd have to wait for his core temperature to come up. He was not too impressed.

There would be occasions when the role of a doctor was liberally interpreted. One wintery night, towards the end of my time in Cambridge Bay, I was awoken by the phone. It was the nurse on call.

"Dr. Dale, there is a report of someone having been killed."

"Well what does that have to do with me? Call the RCMP!"

"They are out of town."

Lynne, the nurse who had phoned me, said that John Lyall was around but he was on his own and wanted help to arrest the killer. John, one of Ernie Lyall's sons, was the local Inuit Special Constable.

"They need you to help bring Mingilgak into custody."

I had a distinct recollection that no job description included arresting suspected criminals! By now I was wide awake anyway so I got dressed and headed over to the little 'matchbox house' where this had taken place. These were tiny, awful houses that had been built as a temporary housing measure some ten years earlier. They were to be used for six months only and then new housing was to be built. In winter they had ice all over the doors and windows. The oil furnaces ran constantly and the Canadian taxpayer covered all heating bills.

That night large quantities of homebrew had been consumed, then a shotgun used at close quarters on Mingilgak's wife. She was quite clearly dead and Mingilgak was standing with a kitchen knife in his hand. There was no shotgun in sight. He struggled a little, so we got him into a snowbank outside. Since he was not dressed well he cooled down quickly and we trundled him off to jail.

Lynne arrived, and she and I went back to the house and had a good look around, trying to figure out what had happened. We moved the body over onto the bed. We had instructions to remain there until the RCMP corporal arrived. This was his case of the year and he burst in, from a party at the Dewline station, and told us not to touch anything. We smiled sweetly and told him that whilst waiting for him, we had rearranged a couple of things! He was disgruntled, but he could hardly complain as it was he who was partying while on call.

Over the following days I spoke with relatives of the

dead woman. There was much talk of revenge. Strangely enough, when the trial took place, they shared my thoughts of sadness over the whole event. It was a crime of alcohol and sociology more than intent. Such were the symptoms of a marginal society. Mingilgak sat in court, looking forlorn and pathetic. Once sober, he had punished himself enough. He received a sentence of two years in jail, then remained over in Frobisher Bay. I met up with him a few years later. I do not know if he ever risked going back to Cambridge Bay.

JULY 20TH, 1975: *I am still trembling somewhat as I enter this in my diary. Today was my closest encounter with death; all due to Bushmills, my dog. Ever since we lived in Burns Lake, this dog had disliked anyone who was inebriated. Earlier today, when outside, he bit into the leg of Steve's trousers. Steve is a tough Inuk hunter, also well known for his drinking propensities.*

I was unaware that this took place, and innocently answered the door, on hearing a commotion outside. I opened the front door to be met with the sight of Steve's shotgun barrel, a couple of feet away from my abdomen. Bushmills was still growling at him, but not biting him. Before Steve spoke I took in the situation and ordered Bushmills to back off, which he did. I got him to go inside the house and then turned back to Steve. The gun remained where it had been, pointing straight at me.

Talking seemed to be a good idea! For, what felt like half an hour, I told Steve what a great hunter he was and what a terrible dog I had, and how there was no doubt that Steve was the best hunter in the community and how he really did not need this annoyance. Steve kept reiterating that he could shoot Bushmills and me. I pointed out to him that if he kept the gun pointed at me, someone would be bound to come by shortly (at least I hoped so), and see him. I told him that this might cause him a lot of trouble with the law, and that maybe he would be sent away to jail. Finally the gun started to lower. It was a double-barrel 12 gauge, and I had not relished the thought of a large hole in my middle.

I promised him that there would be no consequences if he just went home. Shortly after that he left. I will not report it, as it really would achieve nothing but further ill feeling. Afterwards I went inside and poured myself a glass of scotch!

Chapter 11

INFANTICIDE: IMMORAL OR NECESSITY?

JULY 31ST, 1975: GJOA HAVEN. *Clinic finished; Margaret and Ros, the two nurses, are happy and peaceful. I hear classical music playing—Liszt piano pieces—most peaceful. It is very late and I am sitting gazing out over the sea of this natural harbour. Amundsen used it at the beginning of this century. He described it as the "best little harbour in the world." I love Gjoa Haven and often my thoughts turn to that trip in the 'Gjoa' when Amundsen made it through the N.W. Passage. He loved meeting the people here and learned much from them. Important knowledge which he gleaned here helped him on his trek to the South Pole later. The sun is beaming down, out of a cloudless sky, though it is 2 a.m.; the wind is just whistling gently, reminding us of its awesome power here. Down on the beach a woman is carving up a seal, which they caught recently. If I go down to ask her when it was caught, she will answer me:*

"Before."

She is using the 'ulu', a special semi-circular knife, to skin the seal. There is a pervading sense of peace from this timeless scene, which I feel I must somehow assimilate into my soul.

Gjoa Haven has such a delightful harbour, barely below the surrounding land; such a safe harbour, happily used by Amundsen.

In 1908 Roald Amundsen wrote "My Life as an Explorer", which described his successful trip through the

N.W. Passage. He stated then:

"It must, therefore, be the bounden duty of civilised nations who come into contact with the Eskimos, to safeguard them against contaminating influences, and, by laws and stringent regulations, protect them against the many perils and evils of so-called civilisation. Unless this is done, they will inevitably be ruined. All honour is due to the Royal Danish Trading Company for the manner in which it has treated its Greenland colony ... My sincerest wish for the Nechilli Eskimo is that civilisation may never reach them."

Amundsen was certainly sincere, but a dreamer and an idealist. He, like many before him, underestimated the adaptive power of the Inuit. Amundsen was thus, albeit unintentionally, just as much a part of that destructive civilisation which he feared. Later came all the others, worst of all perhaps the missionaries. There are exceptions to every rule, naturally, but by and large there was an arrogance about the presumed superiority of Christianity. Before contact with the whites, the Inuit were quite happily free of guilt and infantile notions of heaven and hell. The Petticoat Lane marketeers of souls deluded themselves into thinking that they were the advance guard of some new civilisation which would help these primitive souls to see the light.

Infanticide was quoted as one example of the primitive and amoral nature of the Inuit. Wiser missionaries studied the anthropology and came to understand a harshly adaptive culture. It is certainly true that the Netsilik Eskimo practiced infanticide, mostly of female babies. This was not done wantonly. One such instance was described to me by a patient at Pelly Bay. I have changed her name as this is a very personal experience. Makkiterk was old and bent almost double from a hard life. She had ten live children. She relayed her story to me:

"One winter had been especially hard and we had not had much to eat in Repulse Bay. My husband tried many times to catch a seal. Many days he stood patiently by the hole, ready with his harpoon, hoping one of the netsik would come up for air at the breathing hole. Sometimes he would wait twelve hours, standing still, bent over, listening intently and watching the tiny little bone; the warning signal. We had no luck and were all very hungry that winter. We got some fish and we stayed in the igloo a lot. Towards the end of the winter we decided to travel to where the Netsilingmiut were camped, somewhere up by what is now called Pelly Bay."

"This journey would take many days but we thought that they might have food and that my husband might catch a seal on the way. Part of the journey would be over land and part over sea ice. We loaded up the komatik, put the children in their caribou parkas and got the dogs ready for the trip. There was only one problem that I could see, and that was that I knew I would have a baby soon. I hoped we could reach Pelly Bay first."

"We set off and the weather was not helping; it blew snow a lot of the way. We did not get any hunting done, so we had to travel on fast as the children were becoming ill by now. Many of the camp we had come from had died that winter and we did not want that to happen to us. On the morning of the fourth day of travel, I began to have pain, so my husband stopped and built an igloo and then left. Soon I had the baby, cut the cord and tied some sinew around it. When all was finished I held the baby for a few moments and cried. My husband had said nothing when he went on and I knew that I had to make a decision. He would accept whatever I decided. I knew that all our lives were in danger now and we had to get to Pelly in a hurry. I had to catch up to my husband and four children really soon.

I put the baby on a piece of fur in the igloo and I left the igloo, blocking up the door as I left. Tears came to my eyes as I walked away. I could still hear the baby crying. After a while, the wind drowned the noise of crying, and my tears stopped. I kept going along the trail and just kept thinking of my family, until I caught up with them. I knew my husband was sad, for we Eskimos love children. We got to Pelly Bay and we all lived."

As she told me this story from forty years earlier, she cried once more. I too, could not hold back my tears and I thanked her for sharing this with me. The Arctic dictates its laws; we have to learn them, respect them and not judge too quickly.

Chapter 12

MEDEVACS AND ARCTIC FLYING

AUGUST 30TH, 1975: CHAR LAKE, VICTORIA ISLAND. *Flew in with Willy Laserich's De Havilland Otter, on floats. Only the second time I get to log hours on this plane. I was able to fly another 1.5 hours on this cumbersome classic plane. Doug Turner is chief pilot and was headed over to Char Lake. I heard that they were going over and contacted Mike Hackman, at Char Lake, to see if he minded a visit. Mike said he would be glad to see me, and soon CF-QQR was in the air. Char Lake camp is at the northwest end of Albert Edward Bay, perhaps forty-five minutes flying time out of Cambridge Bay.*

Recently the Liquor Board had visited Mike, at his camp, and finding no liquor license, had destroyed his liquor. As they prepared to take off, they found that they had a flat battery on their float plane. They had to stay overnight and have dinner with Mike, but sadly, he could offer them no wine!

On the day of our flight, Doug had been hauling char from Wellington Bay, for the local Eskimo co-op fishing industry. He settled into his seat with an accustomed sigh. It had already been a long day. By now it was 8 p.m. and the evening was becoming cool. Doug pulled up the water rudders and pumped the old hydraulic flaps: quick cockpit check; set the prop to fine pitch; wind up the rpm and we were away.

As soon as the stick eased back slightly we were airborne. Otters more or less defy the laws of gravity, flying at surprisingly low airspeeds; we indicated 40 mph on take off. Doug eased the nose down, until we got to a respectable 80 mph, then he handed over to me. I climbed to the grand altitude of 500 feet, but could go no higher, due to snow showers and low scud. We bored through a few clouds. I did not possess an instrument rating but I had read voraciously and practiced whenever I could, so I was safe at the basics. If Doug was not worried then neither was I. Maybe he thought I did have an instrument rating!

Doug was a silent, confident Arctic pilot. He never said anything so I really did not know for sure if I was flying properly. He seemed to be sleeping. We passed Ferguson Lake on the left and then, as we got to Char Lake, he woke up and took over for the landing. Too bad, as I was rather hoping I could do this one. Doug made a long downwind leg to check the water depth and wind, and then we were down.

Climbing up to the camp from the dock, we were met by the Nakasook and Kamoayok children. They were to be picked up for school but they wanted to show us the flies they had been learning to tie. There was a funny old Englishman, who had spent close to $5000 to fly fish for Arctic Char. I tried to talk to him but felt that I had more in common with the children or with silent Doug. I certainly would not tell this English tourist how we hauled Arctic Char out, tail first, after damming a stream!

We had tea and discussed the weather, and what David Kamaoyok Sr. might need next time we were in, then loaded the plane. David had lost both his legs when he was young, from botulism, contracted from rotten caribou meat. Many of his tribe died at that time. His mother had to amputate one of his legs and then he was eventually flown down to the Camsell Hospital, in Edmonton. There the amputations were completed. He was left with wooden legs and never went back for rechecks, fixing them up himself if they needed altering. He became a great hunter but did not like village life and would drink too much when in town. David did like to tease and would sometimes sit in the plane at -40°F with only socks on his feet. Before long someone would get caught and ask him how he could bear it in the cold. He would tell them that he was a tough Inuk, until finally he would laugh and bare his wooden feet!

At 9.30 p.m. it started to get dark so we had to depart. By this time the wind was whipping up an icy blast, so we headed back to the comforts of civilisation. I was able to log another 45 minutes in a Single Otter; every bit helped. We were surrounded by the warm glow of the red lights on the instrument panel. Outside in the gloom it remained sort of VFR flying; some fog was moving in. Doug, as usual, remained unconcerned, and did the landing for me at his usual unhurried pace. The school kids ran off to see their friends and we headed for our warm houses.

SEPT. 2ND, 1975: *On Saturday, Rosie, a Cambridge Bay Inuk, who had given birth a few days before, starts to bleed very heavily. I cannot give her blood as I have none, and have not had the experience or practice at obtaining it at random in the community. I was turned down on my application for O negative blood for emergency use.*

We get the Twin Otter booked and Tug is soon ready for us. We run an IV with Ringer's Lactate and Rosie's husband comes along as well. Oxygen is running of course. On this trip I have to work; no flying. I have to maintain a bimanual uterine pressure, i.e. inside and out, to slow the bleeding. John holds the oxygen on. I fear that she is dead by the time we arrive in Yellowknife; she has virtually non-reactive pupils and is extremely pale. We get her up to Stanton Hospital where she is given O-ve blood immediately! After surgery she does fine, which relieves me greatly. Her haemoglobin was 3 gms before surgery.

After all this excitement, Tug and I had some rum at the Yellowknife Inn and then at 5 a.m. we flew together back to Cambridge Bay via Coppermine. The headwinds were such that we had to fly the longer route. We decided that the co-pilot looked sick, so I informed him that he should sit in the back—I could then log some hours of instrument time legally. If the co-pilot would not agree to be sick, I would threaten him with removal of his medical. Usually, the promise of a beer sufficed. Tug was a hard taskmaster but kinder to me than to his regular co-pilots. At Bloody Falls, he said:

"Can you just take the plane down to 100 feet or even 50 feet, so that I can take some pictures."

He leant out taking snapshots while I flew at 50 feet above the ground. Bloody Falls was the site of the terrible massacre, which took place in 1871, on Samuel Hearne's trip. Later, two priests, Fr. Le Roux and Fr. Rouviere were murdered here.

After we landed at Coppermine we found that the weather was going down fast at Cambridge Bay, so we were stuck. We stayed overnight at the MOT building, making the local cook happy.

"They are a bunch of sparrows here," he explained, "nobody eats a decent meal, so I hope you guys are hungry!"

He happily fed us bacon and eggs, toast and fresh coffee. We walked around Coppermine for a while; then came back for a large lunch; then there was supper.

Coppermine is one of the prettiest villages on the Arctic coast. It is one of the few that were genuine old gathering places. Semi-permanent fishing camps have been there for 4500 years. Coppermine became, many years later, a natural endpoint for explorers. Samuel Hearne, as previously mentioned, was here in 1771 with Matonabbee. From 1913-1916 Diamond Jenness lived here. A member of the Canadian Arctic Expedition led by Vilhalmur Stefansson, Jenness recorded much of the traditional life and produced some wonderful anthropological books and collections of old songs.

By 1948 there was a nursing station in Coppermine. The village was, in early days, larger than Cambridge Bay, but this changed with the construction of the Dewline Station at Cambridge Bay. By 1976 the population of Coppermine was 750. Twice a week a DC-3 or Twin Otter would come in from Yellowknife.

The next day, the weather was fine again and, after a huge breakfast, I logged another 1.2 hours IFR, as we decided that the co-pilot still looked sick! Even on days when the weather is good, there can still be difficulties seeing a horizon in the Arctic. This entails flying on instruments; therefore one often flies 'IFR' even on seemingly good days. In really bad weather, the flying would be known as 'actual' or 'solid' IFR.

We flew over the Coronation Gulf and along the path of Franklin's second expedition to the shores of the Polar Sea. I had examined the area closely before, but today I was working, trying hard to maintain constant altitude and heading. As we got closer to Cambridge Bay I flew in on the VOR, but Tug still did the landing as I was not really supposed to be in the right seat.

The same day we headed straight on to Spence Bay and I began to realize that flying is hard work as I logged another 1.7 hours with 1.2 IFR. Tracking outbound on the 245 ADF I then had to head inbound to Jenny Lind Island, where there was a Dewline Station, manned by a few men who were always happy to chat. We crossed the coast of King William Island and stayed north of Gladman Point, another Dewline Station. Spence Bay had an ADF on 290, which was great as it was hard to find visually. The runway was not great and I admired the skill with which the pilots landed these fairly large planes.

In the winter we would land out on the sea ice. In fact the whole new school was delivered in sections, by a Hercules landing on the ice strip. I was told that Pacific Western landed a 737 jet on the ice but I did not see that.

The population of Spence Bay was 443 by 1976 and there were two nurses. A resident dental assistant was sent up there around 1974. The actual settlement began in 1947 when the Hudson's Bay trader, Ernie Lyall, moved down from farther north. He described the earlier history of that area in his book "An Arctic Man." Ernie was down to earth and pleasantly opinionated, most of the time justifiably. I enjoyed several visits with his family over the years. Spence

Bay, where he lived, is well known for carvings, art, and commercial char fishing.

Later in September I was able to fly actual IFR for almost four hours over to Holman Island and back, with an overnight stay. I learned a great deal of respect for these northern pilots as I became more experienced myself. This helped me in deciding on priorities for medevacs. Tug taught me, patiently, whenever his co-pilots were kind enough to let me take their place. Some of these pilots had ten thousand hours of Arctic flying experience. I had about twenty hours in the Arctic, and a mere 500 in total, at that time.

Tug's son, Mike, flew with him for about three months. It was touching to see a father and son, senior and junior pilots on the same plane. Mike then moved on to DC-3s and finally jets, but the northern experience was great for him. Fuelling up from barrels at -35°F in a wind is a good learning experience for anyone. The passengers even had to help, at times.

Navigation depended on radio aids. Even on good days the ground could be obscured by blowing snow. Tug told me that the majority of their Arctic flying was IFR. Most of the winter is either dark or all white; ground, lakes and sea. Familiarity with the astrocompass was also essential. All neophyte Arctic pilots had to learn this skill and the old pros like Tug and Rocky Parsons made their co-pilots learn their lessons well. Sun shots and celestial navigation were a safe back up. The hours were long and the work tiring but the pilots were appreciated in all the communities they served.

<u>NOV. 20TH, 1975</u>: *Left Gjoa Haven at 1.30 p.m. yesterday with a very sick baby. Communications have been out for a couple of days and the nurse wisely started antibiotics. The baby continued to deteriorate however. When I get back to Cambridge Bay I try to figure out a diagnosis. I do a lumbar puncture and look at the CSF under the microscope. I am not very good at this but the classic pneumococcus has a typical appearance. It is the first time I've seen a pneumococcus; the CSF is cloudy, which is typical of*

meningitis. I am able to find a scalp vein and we start ampicillin IV. Perhaps we won't need a plane tonight. I go home and have a beer but am barely finished when, at 10 p.m. I get a call from the nurses. The IV has gone interstitial. I do not think I will find another—this baby has had previous cut downs for IV's. So now the baby needs to be flown to Yellowknife. One of the nurses wants to go to Yellowknife anyway so there is no point in my going.

I went home tired, hoping for a good night's sleep. The baby was later confirmed as having meningitis but, sadly, was thought to have sustained some brain damage from the infection.

Alas my peaceful sleep did not last long. At 3 a.m. a call came in from Gjoa Haven:

"Dr. Dale there has been a mixed frostbite/burns accident; two Inuit badly injured. Can you get over?"

The problem was that the only plane we had was now well on its way to Yellowknife, with the baby. There was a DC-3 at the Dewline, loaded with thousands of gallons of diesel fuel for delivery. To unload it at the base was apparently impossible in a short time. We had to fetch two stretcher cases from Gjoa Haven, both with IV's running, who would possibly need tracheotomies. Both patients were in shock.

In the end, I arranged for a Mitsubishi MU-2 from Gateway Aviation in Yellowknife, because, on balance, the greater airspeed would make for a faster round trip than taking a DC-3, dumping all the diesel overboard into the sea and flying at 170 mph.

I tried to sleep again, while waiting for the MU-2 to arrive. I was barely asleep when there came another call; this time from Lynne, the Cambridge Bay Nurse:

" John, there is a fire over here!"

Several of us assembled fairly quickly. It was dark and some poor lineman would have to go up the hydro pole to fix a short in a transformer. The short at the top of the pole was starting a fire. The young man who arrived to fix it was already high, from smoking up at a party all night! We sent him higher! It was very cold but he managed just fine. I went back to bed for a while; the plane was not due in until 11 a.m.

After the MU-2 arrived, we hurried over to Gjoa Haven. The Mitsubishi had a global navigation system, which helped to find Gjoa Haven. There was blowing snow and fog all around that day. The flight over was simply beautiful, or perhaps sheer fatigue was inducing a hallucinogenic state. At 18,000' we could see the sun, which was nice as we could not see it on the ground anymore, for the whole winter. A delicate pink bathed everything; the clouds, the engine nacelle, the wing-tip tanks. I tried to pick up some energy from all this beauty. The strip at Gjoa Haven is a couple of miles from town, across the tundra. When we arrived at the nursing station, we found that the nurses had done an excellent job on the patients. IV's were up and running and fluid replacement well under way. Jenny Morris and her fellow nurse were both excellent nurses and had good clinical judgement.

The two Inuit had been out hunting on snowmobiles. Their Coleman stove had exploded in their faces, burning both of them. They then had to snowmobile for several hours in to town. On the way, one was on the sled, just hanging on, but he dragged one arm along on the ground. This one arm had been badly frost-bitten as he had no mitts by then. When we got to Gjoa Haven we dressed the wounds, loaded up the patients and headed off immediately. There was a nurse on board who had come up from Yellowknife. I was almost tempted to take Jenny, as her OR experience might help me more if we had to do a tracheotomy on board.

Luckily the flight went uneventfully and we monitored vitals and fluid replacement until Yellowknife. After landing there, the one Inuk's arm was still frozen solid and made a noise like solid rock when tapped. His neck burns were now starting to cause enough oedema that he needed a trach. Dr. Don Hadley performed this for me, thank goodness. One of the two patients subsequently lost a few fingers; otherwise they did well. Dr. Peter Kallos, a friend of mine from Yellowknife, took the patients on down to Edmonton for further treatment.

Dedication was seen at all levels in cases like this and it was a pleasure to be part of such an effective team. Doctors, nurses, pilots, dispatchers; all may have to give up 24 or 48 hours at a moment's notice. Passengers had their 'sched' flights suddenly changed by us, if we needed the plane. There were rarely complaints at these disruptions.

It was a tremendous boost to me to have friendly treatment at Yellowknife, from my fellow professionals. The invitations to dinner by such friends as Drs. George Gibson, Peter Kallos, Chris Palmer, Ross Wheeler, and Perry Caplan made up for the isolation which I felt very much at times.

From Yellowknife to Cambridge Bay was such a different world that, at times, I did not feel that I had much to talk about with the other doctors. Ross Wheeler had been up visiting and was a little more aware of the strange life I led in the far north. We considered Yellowknife southern civilisation, yet the doctors there helped me by boosting my confidence and giving me telephone advice whenever I needed to call them.

Chapter 13

ISOLATION

Perhaps one of the most isolated jobs in Canada is to be an Arctic doctor in a single doctor post. One of the doctors who had been up to Cambridge Bay before me, Dr. Carl Gill, told me that he felt isolated, lonely and professionally very frustrated. Take a doctor away from his hospital and he has a problem functioning. Most doctors cannot stand being at such a distance from labs and specialists. Doctors who go north challenge their own self-reliance. How well can they function, making serious decisions on their own? There will be no colleague to check with! How many times do we think we have a diagnosis of a 'surgical belly' and then feel much better because we get a colleague to check our opinion? When I left to practice in the south, I always appreciated this luxury, much as I did the luxury of drinking real milk after three years of powdered milk, or seeing the sun in the winter!

In Cambridge Bay the nearest available surgeon was at Yellowknife, six hours away, by plane, in good weather. We had to fly the patient to him first. Some locations had days with no radio coverage. There had to be a high degree of self-confidence and of trust in the strength of the human body, and a certain amount of pure fatalism as well. Dr. Carl Gill exemplified his feelings of isolation with the following case:

"I had this patient with a shotgun chest wound at an outlying settlement. This would have been a straightforward case in Penticton, where I am now; we'd just get help with a chest tube and check blood gases. Up there one had to balance the weather against the state of the patient. I always felt, in spite of the gratitude of the patients, that I could have done more."

To do more, we would need all the surrounding luxuries of a hospital. Dr. Bert Brosseuk, also in Cambridge Bay at one time, and subsequently an internist in the Okanagan, related to me:

"We had a child with epiglottitis in Pelly Bay. The weather went down and although we were sitting right there with a plane, we could go nowhere. Both the pilot, Steve England, and I, felt terrible for many years after. All we could do was try to improve the airway, but the child died."

Nurses, at times, overstayed their period of usefulness in the north. The Northern Health administration was so out of touch with the Arctic that a nurse might cease functioning effectively long before anyone would notice that something was wrong.

On one occasion I had to go to Pelly Bay and physically remove one nurse who had become psychotic. She began to hear voices and suffered from lack of sleep. Being hired directly out of Toronto, and moving into a remote community of 250 Inuit and four whites, was too much for her and being a non-Catholic did not help. This particular community had been over protected by a strong-minded Catholic priest. At the time the regular nurse was a nun.

The young nurse who was sent in, did not stand a chance. The community sided against her, perhaps because she started a relationship with a young local boy. Phone calls at all hours of the night soon caused a psychological break down. I did hear later that she may have had the last laugh, because her young man followed her back to Toronto.

Other nurses, who functioned well but spoke their minds on critical issues, were hounded out of the area by petty minded southern officials.

Sometimes the frustration for the doctor would be in getting details of a case from the nurse. Often the radio and weather combined to make this hard. Telephones were being installed in 1975-1976, but we still relied on radio. The nurses often acted as weather reporters for the pilots, as

RCMP for the police and as general radio operators. Ernie Lyall, who helped a lot in Spence Bay with radio communication problems, remembered one occasion when there was a hepatitis epidemic in Spence Bay. Carl Gill had to travel, by dog-team, from Gjoa Haven; there was no flying, due to the weather. Ernie said it warmed his heart to see the doctor coming in by dog team, just like the old days.

For doctors and nurses the north was a different world. Yellowknife was regarded as a large southern centre, where people could not understand our problems. This could lead to a sort of isolation paranoia, and the wise northern inhabitant kept lots of contact with other kinds of people and travellers. Our problems were, or seemed to be, unique. Only one who had faced similar situations could really understand what was demanded from a person up there. There was a danger of going stale or getting 'bushed', and one had to know when to leave which was not easy. When one became too much of an expert, knew more than fellow workers, looked down on newcomers and wouldn't talk to them, then it was time to go.

For the first few months in Cambridge Bay I enjoyed the new challenge and did not feel the need for colleagues. Gradually the isolation became harder. Cambridge Bay should have had two physicians. There were 2500 people spread over a thousand miles of coast. The area covered was twice the size of Great Britain. I could never give enough attention to Holman Island and Pelly Bay, the more isolated settlements. The nurses had to develop their role as diagnosticians, and some fell into the trap of feeling that they owned the patients. It was hard for them to develop the maturity of a family doctor, who knows his patients will continue to live and break rules as they please, in spite of him. Despite this, the majority of the nurses performed wonderfully, under extremely trying conditions.

Forming cliques was a danger for us all. The community of Cambridge Bay was quite fragmented. I often laughed inwardly at the visiting anthropologists, studying the behaviour of the Inuit when they could equally well have studied the whites! In smaller settlements the wise nurses opened their doors and social evenings to as wide a variety of people as possible.

Blizzards slowed everything down. It would get so quiet, except for the wind, that I would just stay home for days and there was no TV until 'Anik' came in, in late 1975.

In the middle of one blizzard at Cambridge Bay, I got a call from Fred Carnew, the local Superintendent of Education and a personal friend.

"John, can you make it over to my apartment? I have hurt my knee and cannot move!"

The problem was that I couldn't move that easily either. It was not safe to walk far, even in town. The wind was around fifty mph and the temperature near the bottom of the scale. An MOT worker said he would get his Nodwell out. He arrived at my house and we made it down to Fred's. He had a bad effusion on his knee; possibly a ligament tear. I did not think he needed an X-Ray so we strapped up his knee and suggested that he have a glass of whisky!

When we got back into the Nodwell to venture the half-mile home, we drove over a three foot snowbank that had accumulated over the couple of hours we had been there. We did not know if we were on the right track, so we tied string to the door handles and then each ventured out on different sides of the machine until we hit something. This told us that we were still on the road. We drove to the driver's house and then felt the need for some more whisky.

Subsequently I had to walk home. It was not far, but in a blizzard one can get lost right in the middle of a small village. I had to take an angle, off the corner of the school gymnasium, and then maintain that angle to the wind, to get to my house. The biggest problem was for those living in houses on the edge of town. If they missed their house in a blizzard they could wander outside town limits quite easily.

An entry from the diary illustrates, once more, the isolation:

JUNE 12TH, 1976: *Call from Gjoa Haven.*

"John, I think I have a woman with an intra-uterine death."

"How far along do you think the pregnancy is?"

"Thirty-six weeks."

There has been no foetal movement or foetal heart heard for some time actually, so she is certain about the diagnosis. It is midnight. I'm not sleeping anyway. It is summer and total daylight. Later that night she goes into labour. The weather is not great the next day and the woman stays in slow labour. Communications go out and I hear nothing until 2 a.m. the following day, i.e. over 24 hours later. She has arrested in the second stage. I get Gary Butler and Ken Murphy to line up the Twin Otter; they are going on a sched run anyway. I get there at 11 a.m. and start a pit-drip to induce further labour. This runs for about an hour with not much success. By feel I can tell that the position of the baby is head down, or vertex, and that it still might come.

Here is where I wish I was in a nice big hospital where I could ask for help and get an obstetrician to section her. I have to take her out to Yellowknife now. The head is too high for forceps and she is nowhere near fully dilated. At 2.15 p.m. her systolic drops to around 40 mms. Hg. I suspect she has perforated her uterus or has an internal bleed. IV's are set up to replace fluid; we have seven hours of travel before she gets in to Yellowknife, barely conscious. Her pressure has risen to the glorious heights of 70 mms Hg. systolic by this time. We go straight to the hospital and once again stat O negative blood is given, bringing her haemoglobin up. How I wish I could have some blood up there!

After several units of blood she gets much more pain and has the symptoms of a perforated uterus. She is rushed to surgery, has the diagnosis confirmed and gets a partial hysterectomy. The baby was dead, but the mother does just fine. Sometimes it seems nature induces a protective shock mode which, in this case, may have saved her life. I feel responsible for the perforation, because it might not have happened if I had just flown her straight out, after my arrival at Gjoa Haven. I didn't get back to Cambridge Bay until Saturday, 48 hours later.

Another isolation problem occurred when we lost all power at Gjoa Haven; no heat, outside temperature -30° to -40°F. We did not have wood as there were no trees around! Jenny Morris, Lesley Knight, Peter, our 'Jack of all trades', and I, lit up Coleman stoves and tried to keep ourselves warm, and the medications from freezing. Over the next few days the power was on and off. We eventually rigged up an old oil stove; by then the problem was solved and the heat was back on.

Another aspect of isolation was trying to serve two bosses. The southern organization which paid my salary was one boss, but I felt I had an allegiance to the general population up on the Arctic Coast, and in particular to the Inuit. I tried to understand their culture and decide how much of our medical technology to apply. It seemed more important to create a culturally relevant atmosphere for the Inuit, to enable them to determine in what direction things moved, than to be up on the latest antibiotic. I gained few converts amongst the nurses. I tried to get Hugh Brody's book 'The People's Land' as required reading for new nurses but it was a long battle. There is so much medical reading to do that to have someone tell you that you have to learn sociology and anthropology as well can be a nuisance; yet it was essential in dealing with aboriginal peoples.

We were dealing with a society in transition, a marginal culture at the interface of a traditional native culture and a technological civilisation. On occasions I felt that all this fancy medicine, which I had so laboriously learned, was a waste of time. We seemed to be dealing here with some very fundamental political and sociological problems. Those were the times when I was depressed; however, I had been hired as a doctor, not a sociologist, so I had to live with it.

Other doctors before me felt depressed by the impersonal, almost colonial, attitude of the Department. The bosses were all in the south and the problems all in the north. It was frustrating for us to endure the politics. When the new bilingual policy was being implemented, one of the senior doctors in Medical Services hired an MU-2 out of Yellowknife. At considerable cost, he then flew in to every settlement to ensure that the signs outside the nursing station were in English and French. The Minister of Health was due on a tour, and they did not want him to see that the new policy, totally irrelevant in the north, was not being implemented! This same doctor refused to give a ride to one of the nurses they had just fired, on the grounds that she was no longer a Department employee.

To those of us who viewed the plane as a lifeline, often not available when we really needed it, this display of wanton waste was shameful.

Chapter 14

EXPLORERS, ANTHROPOLOGISTS AND PRIESTS

One afternoon in May, 1975, I was riding my Honda 250 XL motorbike near Cambridge Bay, when I noticed an unusual tent down by the beach. On it was written "Japanese Arctic Expedition." Outside, a travel-worn dog team lay resting. Though it was the middle of the afternoon, the occupant of the tent was apparently sleeping; this was not unusual in this part of the world, as everyone ran on their own clocks.

I made discreet noises until a short, heavy set, Japanese man emerged, his face swollen with sunburn. He introduced himself as Naomi Uemura. He spoke very little English, but I gathered that he had just arrived by dog team from Greenland, barely ahead of the ice break-up. Travelling would be hard from now on, especially for the dogs as the ice cuts their paws. By May, leads, or open water spaces, are opening up. Many can still be crossed but it is difficult for the dogs.

During that summer, Naomi followed up on his plan to stay out of town with an Eskimo. In this manner he hoped to learn the language and improve his hunting skills. He picked an elderly man, David, who lived out at Anderson Bay all summer and certainly enjoyed teaching a keen young man and watching him do all the work around the camp!

Naomi was a fascinating throwback to a more romantic era. He was the last person in the world one could imagine selling body and soul to a business life. He escaped this by travelling and writing, and he was a symbol, to many, of the survival of the individual in a society which was becoming increasingly dehumanized.

After University Naomi had started climbing. By 1970 he was internationally known, although most Canadians had not heard of him. He had climbed the highest peaks of five continents; four of them he had conquered alone. The Everest Expedition was with a Japanese team, and was a group effort. He had made the first solo ascent of Mt. McKinley, in Alaska, ultimately to be his burial place. In 1968, Naomi rafted 4,000 miles down the Amazon River in Brazil.

Naomi's interests then turned to the polar regions. A visit to Antarctica led him to develop the notion to go to the South Pole alone. I know that this was his ultimate dream, but there were many hurdles in the way. He went at it with great energy and undertook a 3,000 kilometer dog-team journey, alone, along Greenland's west coast. Then he began the trip on which I met him, during which he followed much of the route of Knud Rasmussen's expedition of the twenties.

After spending the summer out on the land, Naomi returned to Cambridge Bay. Judy and I offered him our house to use as a base, but apart from a meal or two, he did not want to become beholden to anyone. He did not want to lose his acclimatization to the outside, so he lived in his plywood shack on the outskirts of Cambridge Bay until December. By this time it was dark most of the day and often very cold. Once the sea was well frozen and daylight began to return, Naomi could plan the next leg of his trip. He took everything in his stride and had adapted well to the cycle of seasons in the Arctic.

I went out on my skidoo to visit him while he was staying in his plywood shack. The temperature was somewhere around -30° F. There was no heat in the shack and both George Hakungak, my young Eskimo friend, and I were freezing. Naomi lit a smoky fire with driftwood, inside the shack, and we stayed for tea, our eyes running from the smoke. Even George was complaining of the cold by this time, but Naomi had not yet fastened the buttons of his jacket.

Soon after that Naomi headed off for Alaska. He was there by the following spring. Over the next few years I kept track of his travels through friends and I knew that he planned to go to the North Pole first, as a practice run for the South Pole. In a 1983 National Geographic magazine, I read an account of his North Pole trip.

The North Pole had, supposedly, first been conquered by Admiral Robert E. Peary in 1909. In 1969, Wally Herbert, an Englishman, led an expedition from Point Barrow, Alaska, to Spitzbergen which is north of Norway. This was the first trans-Arctic crossing. Naomi, in the spring of 1978, undertook the first solo North Pole trip, considered to be one of the most dangerous journeys ever. He had the help of radio and satellite in pin-pointing his positions. Planes dropped in some of his dog food. Hunting that far north is difficult as there is a distinct lack of game that far from land. A Twin Otter picked him up at the Pole for the return.

Notwithstanding these advantages, Naomi's trip rates as one of the most exceptional solo achievements ever. It requires tremendous determination and courage to travel alone across the Arctic. By constantly battling pressure ridges, the cold, and the open water leads, Naomi was able to achieve his ambition. Once he had to shoot a polar bear that was stalking him, close by his tent. He would travel up to fourteen hours a day, eating mainly at night and cooking with a little kerosene stove.

I knew Naomi was planning his South Pole trip next. Here there were serious logistic problems. The southern regions are controlled by an international agreement formulated by the Scientific Committee for Antarctic Research. Random exploring and adventuring are not encouraged since the whole area is controlled by the agreement. This makes for interesting experiments in working together. On occasions Russian planes have flown sick Americans in to the American air base, but the countries concerned in the Antarctic are not interested in co-operating in dramatic adventures. They prefer serious scientific proposals. Naomi was not interested in that, so he bided his time.

In 1984, I heard the news that a Japanese climber was

lost on Mt. McKinley. It was Naomi. After a suitable search period, he was presumed dead and the search was called off. I felt very sad that such a free spirit had left the world. He remains relatively unknown to the general public in the west, but to my mind ranks as one of the greatest explorers and travellers of all time. I compare him more to Amundsen than to anyone else, because of the precision and thought that went into his travelling. If anyone could havc gone to the South Pole alone it would have been Naomi.

In general, the history of missionaries in the Canadian Arctic is nothing to be proud of; however, I was fortunate enough to encounter several who seemed genuinely dedicated to the well-being of others.

Father Maurice Metayer and Fr. Morice have both been mentioned before. The Oblates have an interesting history. The order of 'Oblates of Mary the Immaculate' was originally founded in Provence, France, in 1815. The members were called the 'Missionaries of Provence' until the name changed to the modern one in 1826. France, just after the Revolution, was in a state of chaos and this order took it upon themselves to improve the situation of the church.

The Oblates came over to Canada in the early part of the 19th century. Bishop Faraud was the Vicar Apostolic for the Mackenzie-Athabasca region from 1832 to 1890. During this time Father A.G. Morice was on his travels in British Columbia. After Bishop Faraud left, a young priest, Breynat, became Bishop in the north at the age of thirty-two. Edmonton had become a base for the Oblates in 1888, and from that centre they began to 'conquer' northern areas.

The Oblates were better funded than the Anglican missionaries. They also cultivated lay-brothers, local members of a native group trained as appointed dignitaries in the church. This gave such individuals status in the community, which helped to produce good public relations. In 1874, when Bompas became Bishop of Athabasca, the Anglicans had only five missions in the area, but the Oblates had eighteen. A race took place to capture the northern primitives to the 'One True Faith'.

This patronizing display of religious colonialism has continued to this day, often misguided yet with good intentions. However, some of the earlier missionaries performed fundamental geographical exploration, Father Petitot being one. Petitot travelled as far as Great Slave Lake and Great Bear Lake, compiling a dictionary of sorts for later explorers to use in their early contacts with Eskimos.

In 1910, Jack Hornby, an eccentric and controversial Englishman, wrote from Dease Bay to Father Ducat at Fort Norman, on Great Bear Lake, suggesting that the priest come and visit the Eskimos. Bishop Breynat sensed that the time was ripe to get as far as the coast and do some converting. He selected Father Rouviere. Hornby was supposed to help, but as usual, was unreliable. Father Rouviere went up to Great Bear Lake and wintered near Hornby, and, in 1911, he made contact with the Eskimos. He describes this first meeting in a letter to his Bishop:

"... I was wearing my cassock and carrying my Oblate cross. This latter strikes them at once. They look at it and I try by signs to tell how he who is on the cross was murdered for us. I shake hands with all of them and give out some medals which I place around their necks. All are overcome with admiration...."

This paternalistic type of encounter between white missionaries and Eskimos was typical of the early days. Things went from bad to worse after that. Father Rouviere seemed a pleasant enough fellow, but soon he was sent reinforcements in the person of Father LeRoux. The younger priest spoke an Eskimo dialect already and would be a useful addition for the journey to the Coppermine Eskimos. LeRoux was irascible and intense and though they worked together during 1912-13, in November 1913 they were both murdered by Eskimos.

In 1916 Inspector LaNauze arrived in the area to determine the fate of the two priests, who had long been reported missing. He eventually arrested two Eskimos,

Uluksuk and Sinisiak, for the murder. It would appear that there had been considerable provocation for the crime, especially by Father LeRoux. The two priests were killed quite close to the already named Bloody Falls. This had been the site of the earlier massacre of Eskimos.

It is possible that the Eskimos thought that priests were supposed to be murdered, like Christ their great leader! After all, Father Rouviere had been showing them the cross and saying how wonderful it was that the one on the cross had been murdered for the human race. Perhaps they thought that they were doing the priests a favour.

After this inauspicious start the Oblates became more cautious in the Arctic. The change from "converting" to "understanding" was a slow process. By the 1960's the Roman Catholic missionaries, at least, were taking a more anthropologically oriented view of Eskimo culture. Other denominations were still involved with converting, and changing the way of life to one arrogantly assumed to be better. A Roman Catholic priest took the lead in helping to establish the Eskimo Co-operatives, which have become a source of tremendous pride to the northerners and also a good source of income for the locals!

Prior to my arrival, in 1974, Father Metayer had been diagnosed as suffering from a cancer in his leg. It had been amputated and he already had an artificial leg when I first met him. I knew him as a patient but we soon became friends; his bookshelf dictated that. In his house in Cambridge Bay there was a sense of timelessness and he and I could discuss philosophy or anthropology endlessly. The house was twenty years old and full of books—most other houses in the community were newer and lacked character.

One day Fr. Metayer came to the clinic complaining of some difficulty breathing, and an X-ray revealed several secondary cancers in the lung. We sought a second opinion but there was not much anyone could do. After that he decided to stay on in Cambridge Bay. Many years of his adult life had been spent here.

I would visit him now as doctor and friend. Our discussions became a little more serious. He wanted to discuss even his own religion it seemed. My lack of belief was not a block to these discussions; perhaps it even gave him greater scope to think freely. He explained to me that his fundamental notion of Christianity was that it was a doctrine of "showing," which fitted fairly closely with my own philosophy of life.

Father Metayer understood my point of view and said that he shared my conviction that a belief which determines action, should be judged by that action. For him it was important to show the inhabitants of the Arctic that there was something of value in Christianity. If they were not convinced by what they saw then it was not for them. He had studied the Eskimos too much and gained far too much respect for their intelligence to make the assumption that Christianity had to be the right religion for everyone in the north. As Wittgenstein's later philosophy stressed the importance of showing meaning in other ways than just words, I appreciated Fr. Metayer's view. The doctrine of showing, as expressed by Wittgenstein, stated a similarly pragmatic viewpoint.

As Fr. Metayer's lungs affected his breathing more and more we were not able to talk as much. I continued to visit him frequently until near the end. One day he seemed anxious, not just in pain. I waited for a while trying to figure out what might be the problem. I knew he was disturbed because his superiors in the order wanted him to go to the hospital at Fort Smith. They felt that he would be more comfortable there. He did not want to go.

Something else seemed to be bothering him that day. I sensed some religious problem. I asked if it was doubts about his faith. He said it was not. Then I realized that it was in some way a fear of death. I could not see why, but on the other hand is not everyone entitled to that fear? I asked him in a subtle fashion if it was this. It seemed to be. We talked about his beliefs.

Fr. Metayer's concept of heaven and hell was not simplistic and it was difficult to follow. There was a sense of self-doubt. He did feel there was an after-life, yet, being so intelligent, had difficulties thinking through the concept. He was somewhat in fear of the whole process of dying. He talked of a peaceful place. I did not say anything very deep or philosophical but he seemed much relieved at the end of that visit. It was perhaps our most important discussion of all. By discussing his faith with a total unbeliever, he seemed to be affirming it. Shortly after that, Fr. Metayer left for Fort Smith to placate his superiors.

Some days later I phoned Fort Smith. I got through to the hospital and to Father Metayer's room. There I spoke to Father Tardy, the priest from Holman Island, who had long been a close friend of Father Metayer. It seemed that Father Metayer had been unconscious all day but during my call he came round and wished to speak to me. He told me that he felt that he was already on his way, and that I would know what he meant from our discussion. He said it felt just fine and all was peaceful. The next day I was told that he had died shortly after our conversation. It was a strange and moving experience.

Chapter 15

CAMBRIDGE BAY TO CAMBRIDGE UNIVERSITY

The last few months in Cambridge Bay were difficult ones. I felt that I had become an 'Arctic Statistic'. My marriage was ending and I was becoming 'bushed'. Being 'bushed', or having 'cabin fever', is really nothing more than a variety of depression. I knew that it was time for me to get out, but I was determined to hang in there until the summer. Then I would be off for a year of study at Cambridge University in England. In the meantime I took as many trips out as I could.

Sometimes paranoia and depression can have give rise to creativity; at other times they may become sinister and morbid and cause a great deal of suffering. There was not only the isolation, but the feeling of frustration which resulted from better communications, but no better understanding of our situation. The innocent and unsuspecting superiors in the south often became the target for all our frustrations. This projection was a necessary survival mechanism. The wiser person would become aware of this and treat it like a game.

The difficult time for me had begun the previous fall:

NOV. 29TH 1975: *Firstly a boredom at all around—a hypercritical state. Then everyone else is personifying all that is least desirable in yourself. THEY drink too much etc. Following this a sad realization that this may all be your own fault: it's the way you see it. You have changed and your outlook has become narrow, self-centred, depersonalized; in fact you can't hack it anymore. If someone phones and says come on over, you just can't see the point.*

I feel like a zombie—moody, subdued, depressed, bitter, cynical. In fact I am probably well and truly bushed. This will not be solved by a short break outside, because the central problem is my own inability to live with myself. Perhaps being bushed is a fundamental personality problem, triggered by some event. It is not some psychiatric illness that can be neatly classified. I will have to come to terms with an inner self, find hidden strengths.

In retrospect I should have left the Arctic earlier. There was some masochistic tendency to hang on and think I could solve something by staying longer. Away from Cambridge Bay itself I could still relax with various Inuit friends. This was the time of the murder, after which I had to help arrest the killer. I was not enjoying the job or Cambridge Bay anymore, due to my personal circumstances, yet I did not want to leave before my target date. Hanging on is what it was that last summer. What friends I did have were important, as were duck hunting trips and ice fishing expeditions.

I finally left in August of 1976 and flew to England, allowing some time to find a place to stay for the year at Cambridge. The initial adjustment to Cambridge University was hard for one who had become used to saying "yes" with his eyebrows and "no" with his nose! I felt like T.E. Lawrence, in the movie "Lawrence of Arabia," when he was so awkward, on his return to Cairo, trying to be 'English' once more.

That summer was the beginning of a whole year away from medicine, in order to study Polar Regions. I had ulterior motives to be at Cambridge. I wanted to catch up on my studies of Bertrand Russell and Ludwig Wittgenstein. This was the place, after all, where they both studied and taught. Russell first went there in 1890, then developed with Alfred Whitehead, 'Principia Mathematica', a work which tried symbolically to derive mathematics from logic.

In 1912, Wittgenstein became Russell's pupil and Russell was convinced that he was teaching a genius.

During the First World War, Wittgenstein was in Austria and Italy, and was captured by the Allies. He and Russell met later to discuss Wittgenstein's first book. That led to a parting of the ways and they related only superficially from that time on. Wittgenstein eventually came back to Cambridge, as a lecturer, in the late twenties, but did not publish another formal book until close to his death in 1964. I took in as many philosophy seminars as I could during that year at Cambridge.

The Scott Polar Research Institute had been founded in 1920 as a memorial to Captain Robert Scott of Antarctic fame. He had died, in March 1912, on the return from the South Pole. At the Pole he had found, to his dismay, that Roald Amundsen had beaten him to that prize. Antarctic explorers Frank Debenham and Sir Raymond Priestley had later founded the Institute and it has grown to be an international mecca for Polar Studies.

Within the University the Institute is a centre for teaching and research. Subjects covered there are as diverse as geology, anthropology, physics of sea ice, oceanography, glaciology, and the history of Polar Exploration. One can find experts on almost any topic of relevance to the Arctic or Antarctic. I felt humbled, as I had never considered that I was an academic, neither did I consider myself an Arctic expert, yet we were all made to feel that we had something to offer to the Institute.

The permanent staff were of the highest calibre and very excited by their work. This was contagious. Dr. Gordon de Q Robin was the Director at this time. His interest was in glaciology but he seemed interested in all aspects of Polar Research. Five post-graduate students had gathered to spend the year writing theses. We wrote on such diverse topics as:

"The Tectonic Evolution of Antarctica."

"Psychological illness amongst Canadian Eskimos."

"The role of Deception Island in the development of Antarctic affairs."

"Psychological aspects of group behaviour in Antarctica."

"Eskimo Bowhead Whaling in Alaska."

Visiting Cambridge that year was Dr. Joe MacInnis from Canada. Joe was there researching a book and later went on to produce many television specials in Canada. He also organized diving expeditions to the 'HMS Breadalbane', a sunken ship in the Arctic. There were many other visiting experts, such as Wally Herbert, who had travelled across parts of Greenland, and to the North Pole, by dog-team.

There was a seminar with Sir Vivian Fuchs, who, together with Sir Edmund Hillary, had led the Commonwealth Trans-Antarctic Expedition in 1955-1958. Hillary went from one side of the continent laying in depots for fuel, using Ferguson tractors and aircraft support. He then made it to the Pole and returned back to his base. Fuchs crossed from the other side and then continued on in Hillary's tracks. The top of the interior plateau is 10,000 feet above sea level, so there are many altitude and terrain problems in addition to the expected rigours of polar travel.

Another seminar was with Hugh Brody. I had read his book whilst in the Arctic and had a high opinion of his abilities. He had lived for almost two years with an Inuit family in the Pond Inlet area of Baffin Island. He subsequently recounted his experiences in "The People's Land." This study of the modern Inuit has become a classic in its field.

I sat in the back of the class at Dr. Ross Harrison's philosophy lectures whenever I could. His lectures on epistemology were manna to my jaded brain. I was able to attend several seminars chaired by Peter Winch and John Wisdom. Professor Stefan Körner came to lecture on one occasion. I had read books by most of these people and it was exciting to see them in person. Unfortunately Con Drury, my old mentor, died during that year and I did not get to see him again. He had followed with such interest my time in the Arctic.

During that year I also discovered a flying club which rented Tiger Moths! The De Havilland Tiger Moth was a famous old biplane, so I had a two hour checkout and was then free to roam the countryside of Cambridgeshire with scarf and goggles. This was an open cockpit biplane, with a 120 H.P. Gypsy Moth inverted-six engine. The two mag switches were on the fuselage outside and the prop was hand swung for starting. There was no canopy, no brakes and no tailwheel. My father had taught on these and so had an uncle, both in the Royal Air Force. For me it was nostalgic.

Take-off was at 45 mph then climb at 65 mph. Normal cruise was 85 mph and "never exceed speed" was an incredible 170 mph! This meant that it was good for aerobatics. As soon as my checkout was finished I was able to head off and have fun. I thought I saw the instructor winking when he said no aerobatics approved.

In no time I was happily looping and spinning with the old biplane. I had to land on the grass as the airport manager did not want the runway torn up by the tail skid. If you had a passenger you had to communicate with a rubber Gosport tube. It worked quite well; the radio didn't. The weather could be a challenge with an open cockpit. In one rainstorm I was severely lashed by rain, which felt like small bullets on my face, but this was part of the romance of open cockpit flying!

The year drew to an end. I finished my thesis and was examined on it, then went off to Greece on a motorcycle for a couple of weeks. It was a BMW 1000 cc. R100RS; an enjoyable way to travel in Europe and a great end to the year.

Chapter 16

NANISIVIK, BAFFIN ISLAND

In August, 1976 I headed back to British Columbia, taking the BMW with me. I visited with my sister, Janet, in Vancouver, and did some touring around B.C. on the motorbike.

Within a short period of time I received a phone call:

"How would you like to go to Baffin Island?"

I gave this considerable thought. I was now single and knew what to expect up north. It might be even harder to take. I felt recovered from all the annoying feelings at the end of my time in Cambridge Bay. On the other hand, I had read so much more now of the history and here they were offering me Nanisivik a mining town at the north end of Baffin Island. This was another whole area of the Arctic which most people never get a chance to see in their entire life. I had to go! I took a flight from Vancouver to Montreal and on up to Frobisher Bay, now known as Iqaluit. A two week orientation in Frobisher was followed by a 700 mile flight to Nanisivik, by Twin Otter.

Nanisivik was a different kind of settlement for me; primarily a transposed mining company town. Some of the nearby communities were among the most beautiful in the Arctic; Grise Fiord and Pond Inlet being two of these. This far north it was truly "the land of the midnight sun" and, in winter, it was dark from November until March.

There were 250 inhabitants at Nanisivik and there was a contract stating how many Inuit had to be hired and trained, but there were still many more whites than I had been used to. There were seventy Eskimos and the mine had been running for almost two years at this time. There was supposedly some kind of a contract guaranteeing the presence of a local doctor. There had never been one up here before and there did not seem to be much need.

During my time there I did have to attempt a tooth extraction on an Inuk, an acquaintance from Cambridge Bay. Eddie Kikoak wanted me to take his tooth out, to save himself a trip to Frobisher Bay, a long way south. I explained to him that I had never pulled out any teeth before. He did not seem worried by that. He drank most of a bottle of whisky before he arrived, and I duly attempted to remove the offending tooth. Unfortunately it broke just below the gum line so I had to tell Eddie that he would still have to take his trip south.

A few days later fate had its revenge; I had an infected root canal! I had to wait for the next plane south and go down to Frobisher Bay. There, a well meaning young dentist informed me that I would have to have several appointments over at least two weeks. This meant staying in the 'Hotel' in Frobisher. This was about as aesthetic as staying in jail, so I went back the next day and to the dentist's horror told her to pull my tooth and let me worry in the future about bridging it. She was not impressed, but I did not know anyone in Frobisher and the thought of two weeks in a hotel there was more than I could stand.

The whites in Nanisivik felt reassured that there was a local M.D. The mine was unusual in that it offered a family package with guaranteed employment for spouses and good day-care for children. The need was more for the psychological assurance of having a resident doctor. In fact it was not such a bad idea, as the nurse was totally 'bushed'. She had been on her own far too long but my pleas to have her removed fell on deaf ears down south.

This same nurse locked herself inside the nursing station for several days. Neither I nor anyone else in the community could get in. There were no emergencies, so I discussed the situation with the local RCMP and we decided to leave her there. We played cards for several days and ate gourmet meals as Neil Davidge, the local RCMP officer, was a good cook. Northern Health were unconcerned with the situation. The nurse eventually opened the nursing station again and life returned to normal. I made sure I had a key after that!

I settled in, played badminton, and usually listened to 'Morningside' on the CBC, watched the one channel on TV, and read philosophy for about four months. There was very little work to do. I enjoyed visits to Arctic Bay, a nearby community, with Neil Davidge. This entailed a twenty mile drive, which was pleasant in good weather, otherwise sometimes a challenge.

There was not enough travel for me, and the Frobisher doctors fought over opportunities to serve the outlying communities. I felt already that there was a new kind of doctor in the north. I had studied, by now, enough sociology and anthropology to realize that medicine was just a small part of a political and cultural milieu. The doctors whom I met were able technicians but did not seem to be so interested in the broader picture.

The excitement of the Arctic was still with me, and I would have loved to have seen the summer there; however I began to feel that my medical skills were being eroded. After four years of experience in the High Arctic, I did not feel like settling in Yellowknife and decided to go further south, to British Columbia. It was time to be an ordinary doctor and to regain some lost skills. I had not treated one heart attack in the last few years and had seen only one case of diabetes. The Inuit did not have stomach ulcers, but cancer seemed to have a normal occurrence rate. Eskimos also did not fuss about minor ailments to the same degree as did people in the south. I would have to get used to all that again! I quit the job in Nanisivik in December of 1977 and headed back to British Columbia.

I knew that I would still want to make trips to the Arctic. This would mean getting an aeroplane. The love of the north stayed with me and I was lucky enough, later, to own a private aircraft. This gave me the opportunity to travel north.

Chapter 17

RETURN TO THE ARCTIC

Immediately following my move from Baffin Island to B.C., flying took an even larger role in my life. It had been six years since I had owned a plane. I took some extra training in psychiatry in Toronto while I finished up my Commercial and Instructor ratings and I then flew 'bush' planes commercially for a short time, back in British Columbia, before going into full-time practice again. As the Arctic passion remained, I had to fly myself back up there whenever I could. To fly to the Arctic, in a small private plane, is not a light undertaking but I did have an advantage in having some experience. However, flying a Twin Otter, right seat, with a highly experienced pilot in the left seat, is different from flying a small four seater. I had to decide what kind of a plane to buy, bearing in mind the dream to return north.

A minimum range of 400 nautical plus reserve is safe. Greater range provides more peace of mind for northern flying. At the time of my first private trip back to the north, in 1981, I flew a Maule M5-235, powered by a Lycoming O-540, with 235 HP. This was a great plane for this kind of flying. I had dreamt, for many years, of owning a Maule.

There are different routes that one can take to fly to the Western and Central Arctic. Whitehorse and north is one possibility, unfamiliar to me. Going straight north from Prince George and Fort Nelson, via Fort Simpson and the Mackenzie River, is a good route to Inuvik and Tuktoyaktuk. I was familiar with this route. Two routes go north from Yellowknife, one via Contwoyto Lake, with refuelling there from carried gas, the other via Great Bear Lake. Port Radium, on Great Bear Lake, makes a good refuelling spot, as long as one has extra gas in the plane, as there is no gas available there. If a plane can safely make Coppermine or Cambridge Bay with good reserves then one can go direct. Reserves should not be the usual forty-five minutes of gasoline, as in the south. They should be based on where else one might have to go if the weather should change drastically.

Navigation is simple nowadays with GPS (Global Positioning Satellite), so that has solved one major problem. However, since the late eighties, the Dewline Stations have closed and that has shut down a major safety communications network, previously available to the private pilot. The tundra looks inviting to land on but is boggy and rough when seen from closer range. Any four-seater aeroplane had better be considered a two-seater for Arctic flying. Survival gear, spares, extra gas and warm clothes take up a lot more space than usual.

On my first return trip north, in 1981, I took the Maule and went first from 100 Mile House, British Columbia, to Yellowknife. Echo Bay Mines had given me permission to land at Lupin/Contwoyto Lake. My partner and I headed up that way, landed there and put in our own fuel. Later they sent me a $200 landing fee which I refused to pay. After take-off, I stayed too low, lost my ADF coverage and wandered off course. This was on the same routing that had caused Martin Hartwell to become lost, in bad weather. The only ADF beacon, or NDB as they are otherwise known, was near Contwoyto Lake.

Eventually, by reading the next WAC map, I found I had wandered off to the east. I flew straight north, to pick up a coastline, and eventually made it into Bathurst Inlet. Then I had to wait for someone to come over from the lodge so that we could go back with him, in the boat. An Inuk, Henry, who recognized me immediately from my last clinic there six years earlier, was the one who boated over for us. Once at Bathurst Inlet Lodge, we filled our gas cans, paying a very high gas price, as we expected. The strip at Bathurst is not for the unprepared; in fact I would not recommend it for small planes at all. My landing there was not by choice. It is tundra and better suited to Twin Otters or DC-3s. Strangely enough, the Flight Supplement says the same thing! It was safe in the Maule but it was a true soft field landing and take off.

We were invited by the owner of the lodge to stay overnight. The next day he added a considerable overnight fee on top of the gas price. I would not have stayed if I had known that, as it was daylight all the time, and we could have flown on to Cambridge Bay at any time of the day or night. Going in to Cambridge Bay we got the ADF at 8000' and 180 miles away. It is good to know where you are going up there!

As we crossed the Coronation Gulf, the Dewline had us on radar at 7000' and helped us in. Cambridge Bay had good runways for almost any plane, gravel, but well packed. Fuel is expensive up north but it is good to try and check ahead, as there are some airports where the price is exceptionally high. On the ground at Cambridge Bay, the next critical thing for a small aeroplane was the tie-down. There is always the likelihood of a good blow, even a blizzard, so aircraft tie-down is important. Overnight accommodation in most Arctic settlements is expensive and, if one is on a budget, the choices are tenting or making some arrangement with a local family.

After we landed at Cambridge Bay, we went into town and met up with old Mahik. He found us a place to put sleeping bags down for the night and invited me out fishing. The Arctic char run was on and soon we were latching onto five to twelve pounders in the nearby river mouth. After a few days at Cambridge Bay, we took advantage of the safety network of Dewline Stations and flew east, over to Gjoa Haven. From Cambridge Bay east, across Jenny Lind Island, was just over 200 nautical miles, with nowhere to land in between. This meant flying directly across the bleak coastline where all Franklin's crew had perished. Looking from 1000' above, the terrain was distinctly unfriendly; rock and shale, with little vegetation and no signs of animal life. This is the flat part of the Arctic. The Non Directional Beacons were plentiful because of the Dewline Stations, so navigating, once up here, was easy. Getting up here was the hard part!

At Jenny Lind Island, the Dewline operator was happy to chat with us before passing us on to the Gladman Point operator. Gjoa Haven is only fifty miles farther and we landed on a new runway, built since I was last there. The runway was now 4400' long at 150' above sea level; however, it still seemed as though there was always a crosswind for landing. The runway was wide enough to make a diagonal landing, to try to get into the wind. At Gjoa Haven it was harder to find a good tie-down, but we made do with some gas barrels. The tail wheel tire blew on landing, but an old friend, Andy Polangniak, was able to help me fix it in no time.

The settlement of Gjoa Haven is two miles south-west of the runway, but if a plane lands, locals will soon arrive in three-wheelers or whatever.

After Gjoa Haven it was a short hop over to Spence Bay. We had a passenger from Cambridge Bay, an Inuk boy whose uncle was working at the Shepherd Bay Dewline Station. After permission was granted from Denver, Colorado, we were allowed to land at the Dewline Station. Ambrose Aknavigak was there to meet his nephew. Ambrose was Mahik's son. After we arrived, the weather turned foggy, so we stayed overnight and ate like kings. It was, however, sad to see that the same 'institutional syndrome' still existed at the Dewlines. Some residents liked to talk to newcomers; others just passed you in the station without any greeting.

Ambrose wanted to fly over to Spence Bay and visit relatives. I thought that was great, as we had been lucky enough to stumble on some free gas at Gjoa Haven, and wanted to fly as much as possible. Ambrose did weigh around 260 pounds, so with four on board we needed all the horsepower we could get! We were at sea level so it was fine. By taking Ambrose we automatically had an overnight place to stay at Spence Bay, and Pat Lyall, Ernie's son found me some gas. When it came time to take Ambrose back the next day, fog had settled in. We took off with a 250' ceiling but were on instruments in no time and, as I was not legally rated, we turned back, got below the fog and landed at Spence Bay again.

By the next morning the weather had improved. We dropped Ambrose back at Shepherd Bay and headed over to Gjoa Haven, for the last of the free gas, before departing for Cambridge Bay. Fern, the radio operator from Shepherd Bay, was worried about our small private plane and kept updating me on the weather. He came on the radio:

"Quebec Juliet Delta, Shepherd Bay: Cambridge Bay latest is 3000' overcast, wind 090 degrees, 25 knots, gusting to 35."

This was not bad weather, except I would have liked to have crossed between King William Island and Victoria Island at a higher altitude. Flying over water, in a land plane, always worries me. The water and floating ice looked cold and unfriendly. A few minutes later the radio came on again:

"Hey, is that John Dale?"

"Affirmative, who is calling?"

It turned out that one of the pilots who used to fly Twin Otters out of Cambridge Bay, Gary Butler, was just passing overhead in a Nordair 727 Jet. He was now right-seat pilot in this plane, and from their position could give me the altitudes of the cloud layers. This enabled me to ascend through some cloud and pass over the sea at a higher, safer altitude. Then all I had to do, closer in to Cambridge Bay, was to let down through some snow to an altitude from which I could see the ground. We came out below cloud at 1000', in light snow, precisely as Gary had said we would. The Cambridge Bay radio operator came on at that time:

"Wind at 90° to the runway at 25 knots gusting to 35."

She then gave me the option to land wherever I wished, adding that a Twin Otter ahead of me had just had a hard time with the wind. I landed across the runway at the taxiway exit. We stopped in 100 feet! This time the plane was tied down with more care than usual, in light snow and 30 knot winds.

Leaving Cambridge Bay the next day, we flew via Tree River to Coppermine. The coast there has rolling hills and lush grasslands. It looks deceptively as if one could land anywhere; yet on the tundra, landing can be treacherous. Tundra, in the brief summer, turns into a soft spongy, wet surface. Landings are only possible on eskers, the raised beds of shale left by ancient glacial rivers.

The terrain around Coppermine is, nevertheless, far more hospitable than that of the northern islands. After landing there, we threw up the tent and made supper. Shortly after, Keith Crowe, the author of "A History of the Aboriginal Peoples of Northern Canada," walked over and we chatted for a while. The evening showed off the Arctic at its very best. The sun stayed bright and it was warm there compared to Cambridge Bay. On the previous day it had reached over 80°F. The late evening sun cast long shadows; there was not a breath of wind, and not a cloud in the sky. It was a pleasure for me to meet someone whose book I admired, and to share such a beautiful evening with another who loved the Arctic.

Bev Brooks was the local radio operator. She invited us to join her on a fishing trip, after her shift. This would be at 2 a.m. We fished until 5 a.m., out in the ocean, and caught whitefish. We finally slept at 6 a.m. Later that same day we left, flew via Bloody Falls once again, and headed down to Port Radium on Great Bear Lake. Port Radium had come into its own as a uranium mine during the early part of the war. The runway was 5000' long but had some nasty downdrafts on the one end.

At Port Radium we were able to cook lunch and gas up with the extra gas purchased at Coppermine. The rest of the trip, via Fort Simpson to Dawson Creek, was uneventful; by then we were flying on the magnetic compass. At Dawson Creek we took the time to go into town for Chinese food. Our only good food on the trip had been the at the Dewline Station!

Chapter 18

TUKTOYAKTUK

My second trip back to the Arctic in a small plane was in May 1985. Bob Miller and I decided to head up and take a look at the Inuvik-Tuktoyaktuk area of the Beaufort Sea. Bob was an ideal travelling partner, having been a trapper, in the Blue River area of B.C., for most of his life. The original plan was to try an early season trip to Tuktoyaktuk, go on to Holman Island and then visit an old friend in Coppermine.

With the Maule stripped of its back seat and loaded up with survival gear, snowmobile suits, rifle, tent and more, we were ready to go.

Take-off, out of 100 Mile House B.C. on May 3rd, was accompanied by the usual cross wind, and we could feel the load on the plane. North of Prince George, we hit major turbulence and had to slow the plane to 16 inches of manifold pressure and 120-125 mph. We stopped overnight at Dawson Creek, waking up in the morning to miserable weather. We could only creep, in marginal VFR (Visual Flight Rules) weather, into Fort St. John which was quite close by. We had hoped to make Tuktoyaktuk on that day. Lloyd Olsen, at the Esso dealership, loaned us his car and we were able to go into town for some decent food.

On May 5th, we were able to depart to the north. There were clouds at 7500' broken, so we went above that until it became solid cloud cover. At one point, when we had to go on instruments for a brief spell, I noticed that my artificial horizon instrument was failing. This was not fun! The artificial horizon is probably the single most critical instrument that a pilot needs to stay safe when flying without ground reference. Fort Nelson had a 1500' ceiling so we gassed up and headed north. Fort Simpson was below limits, so we bypassed it and kept on up the Mackenzie, stopping at Wrigley. Enroute, we received weather assistance from an American Airlines jet, up at 35,000'. The pilot kindly passed on my intentions to Fort Simpson. From Wrigley on, the cloud ceiling was 1000', forcing us to stay at 500' all the way up the river to Norman Wells. The artificial horizon seemed to be working again, which was a relief as it was likely that I would be needing it later. The weather in the Arctic can be unpredictable.

As we hurtled along low and fast, we passed the occasional Indian family camped beside the river. The ice was opening up and we could not land on the river in an emergency. At 500' above ground there was not a lot of time to pick a landing place anyway.

We were longing for the safety of good solid ice, farther north. As we flew closer to Norman Wells, the radio operator informed me that a large snowstorm was inbound for the airport and he would have to close it soon. There was no way we could return south; we did not have enough gas. Within ten minutes I could see the storm ahead and our narrow tunnel began to close up. I opened the Maule to full power and 160 mph, and the ceiling lowered to 700' with visibility 2-3 miles ahead. As we landed, we were enveloped in snow, and the operator closed the airport officially, having stretched the shut-down time so that we could land.

The weather stayed unpleasant, but we were lucky enough to be offered sleeping bag space by the local helicopter pilot. Eight dollar greasy cheeseburgers had to do for supper! Norman Wells was like an old ramshackle instant frontier town. It was literally built on oil in 1911. The first well was drilled in 1919. By 1944, there were 64 wells and the Canol Pipeline was built, for the war effort. This pipeline ran to a temporary refinery in Whitehorse. It was dismantled after the war, but another one, which ran as far as Alberta, was opened later.

When we woke up the next morning, the weather looked fine. In Tuktoyaktuk it was '1/2 mile visibility in fog';

however Inuvik was open, and had to be a nicer place than Norman Wells! We took off and flew, in beautiful sunshine, over to Inuvik. It was one of those days which made us realize why we had come north. A blanket of pure white snow covered the ground; the brightness of the sun's reflection forced us to wear sunglasses. As we flew, a sense of exhilaration and excitement overtook us, and we now felt as if we were getting into the true north. Certainly I had trepidation, for I had never flown in this part of the Arctic and it was early in the year. Choosing this season was a deliberate decision, because the sea ice would be solid. We wanted to fly out to the oil rigs and land on the ice wherever we could.

After landing at Inuvik, there was a demand on my professional skills. Some unfortunate fellow was convulsing; my first clinical guess was that it could be from alcohol withdrawal. That suspicion was confirmed. After he had settled, I was surprised by a familiar voice:

"Well look who's here, grabbing the limelight as usual!"

I turned around and bumped into Mike Tugwell, whom I had last seen at Cambridge Bay. Mike was now flying a Chevron Hawker-Siddely 748 and also the company Cessna Citation jet. We visited for a couple of hours and then headed over to Tuktoyaktuk, as there was a window in the weather. These 'windows' have to be grabbed as opportunities. The weather can change in a matter of minutes, and we had heard that the fog bank had just moved five miles out to sea.

The flight was only forty-five minutes, but by now we were beyond the tree-line and I had to concentrate on my navigation skills. We were still dependent on VOR and ADF navigation but both needles were 'alive' into 'Tuk'.

Approaching Tuktoyaktuk, we called, on the Beaudril company radio, to alert Carter Kelly that we were about to land. Carter was in charge of airport logistics for Beaudril. Coming closer to 'Tuk', I realised how easy it would be to miss this whole village, in bad weather; something we were to think about more seriously later on. Carter was there to meet us and we had to go and make the tie-downs. These northern airports were not accustomed to small planes that needed to be protected against the ever present high winds.

Bob and I unloaded all our gear, except the booze; this was a dry community, so the rum had to remain on the plane as survival gear! I had been able to arrange an invitation to stay at the Nalluk Base belonging to Gulf Oil. I had wanted to compare the modern industrial Arctic with the Arctic I had known several years earlier. Nalluk Base was luxurious and we were soon installed in our quarters.

We first wanted to explore Tuktoyaktuk itself. 'Tuk' was in earlier days known as Port Brabant. The Inuktitut name translates to 'Looks like a caribou', and the older village, nearby, was known as Kittigazuit. Historically this was an unusual village in the Arctic, in that there were perhaps 1000 Inuit living there as long ago as 900 A.D.

Kittigazuit was an example of a Thule culture village and would have been a semi-permanent whaling settlement. It existed for several hundred years; as long as there was a plentiful supply of whales. Bowhead whales and right whales were numerous until the seventeenth century, when serious hunting, using whaling ships, began. After that time it became impractical for the Inuit to remain year round in the village. The 'Little Ice Age' may have been a further reason for the abandonment of semi-permanent housing. Igloos and dog-teams have become common only in the last few hundred years, probably as the Inuit were forced to become travelling hunters.

Dr. John Richardson, visiting this area in 1826, reported several villages in the area around Kittigazuit, Cape Bathurst and Atkinson Point. By the end of the 19th century, the lack of resistance to introduced diseases was taking its toll. The Karngmalit Eskimos were reduced from 2000 to 20.

Tuktoyaktuk, by 1985, numbered about 900 locals, with an interesting mixture of backgrounds. Also by 1985, there were several hundred oil company employees present at any one time. The oil companies made every effort to protect the locals from harmful influence, but contact was unavoidable.

The new company 'palaces' were awe inspiring to one, like myself, used to 'honey buckets' for toilets and no TV. Even telephones seemed a luxury in the Arctic. The infamous 'honey bucket' was a garbage bucket, sized to take a toilet seat and a cover. The inside was lined with a standard heavy duty garbage bag of the black indestructible variety. As it neared full, there was always a battle to avoid having to take it out. A 'twistem' was applied and the whole disgusting thing would be thrown outside in a 45 gallon garbage pail. A most unsanitary arrangement! Hepatitis outbreaks were not uncommon until a better system replaced all this.

At Holman Island I had heard a tale that an eager hunter, out on the sea ice, had stalked a black seal only to find, as he closed on it, that it was a 'honey bag'. Those of us in luxury houses had septic tanks, which were tanks stored in one part of the house so that they would not freeze.

Staying at Tuktoyaktuk—at Nalluk Base—was luxurious, but a striking contrast to the Arctic I knew. Our quarters were the guest suite; two bedrooms, private living room, kitchen and bathroom with shower. There were 200 people on the base, and the place was equipped with a steam room, jacuzzi, sauna, exercise gym, and squash court. There were TV rooms, video game rooms, snooker rooms; even a reading room, but very few books. A cafeteria, open 24 hours with free food, was only outclassed by the main dining room. Here one ate cordon bleu meals. As we were weathered in here we had no choice but to sample all this food! I needed a squash game every day to avoid ending up looking like a beluga whale.

There was, however, a certain sense of frustration about having come all this way to experience an artificial community, and then to sit inside gazing at the Arctic outside. I felt trapped here. Here I was, in this climate-controlled environment, feeling frustrated. I could walk outside, but I did not feel I was a part of the Arctic. The residents at the base feared the locals and told us that if we went to town we would run the risk of being knifed. The Inuit, we were informed, were totally unpredictable when drunk.

Our culture seemed to be redefining the Arctic. It was now simply something to be conquered and profited from, not experienced. We were no longer willing to learn from the Arctic. It was time to show it mastery—time to show our superior culture. I felt sad and confused by all that I saw around me in the bases.

Arriving in Tuktoyaktuk on May 7th, we found the weather forecast to be looking unfriendly for the next few days. Jim Guthrie, the base manager, was to go to Herschel Island by Twin Otter the next day, and asked if I would like to join him. As the weather was below my limits, I thought that it would be a good learning experience to accompany the Twin Otter pilot. The ceiling was 300'—400'. We climbed out and went on top at 4000', a luxury unavailable to me as I did not have an instrument rating

I remembered that this had been the place where I had slept so often, during my previous time up north. Often, sitting in the marginally comfortable seats of a Twin Otter had been my only sleep in days. The drone of the two engines would lull me off in no time. On this occasion I fell asleep soon after we were above the clouds. Soon, homing in on a company ADF beacon, we let back down and landed on the sea ice. There were plenty of seals and some fairly rough ice, then an airstrip near the 'Munaksee', a warehouse ship. The ceiling was 150', but that was all in a day's work for the pilot. Selby Wiseman, from Newfoundland, met us at the home-made airstrip and drove us over to the ship. This particular ship is a floating warehouse and used to carry railway box cars on built in tracks, between Seattle and Alaska.

Enroute to the Munaksee' we stopped to watch a seal. He was quite unconcerned by our presence, and I was able to walk up to within four feet of him. In my earlier experience here he would have been on the supper table, but we would never have managed to get that close. The seals were protected and even fed near here, but not the polar bears. They were shot. Each ship maintained an Inuk, armed, to keep marauding polar bears at bay. On board, we had a very pleasant lunch and then drove over to the 'Gulf

Beaufort', a floating gas station.

Other sundry ships and a rig were frozen in around here. There was no open water yet and the ice was still good. Nearby stood the 'Kulluk', a conical semi-submersible drilling unit. A versatile tool, this was used to drill in 600' of water and at that time was awaiting the break-up of the ice. Ice-breakers were frozen nearby. The 'Kalvik' and the 'Terry Fox' were both here, in addition to a couple of supply vessels. The overall appearance was that of a busy place. It lacked only traffic lights and an air traffic controller. There were roads hither and thither, named and with intersections; all on the sea ice. Once again, I was in another world!

Okanagan Helicopters had a Bell 212 working here and Pat Casey and John Morris were the pilots. Pat called me after we had finished wandering around:

"How would you like to go over to the 'Moliqpaq'?"

I did not need to be asked again. The 'Moliqpaq' was the most interesting rig up here. We flew over at the customary helicopter altitude of 500', looking down upon solid ice interspersed with open leads of water. Landing up on the 5th deck, on the heliport, we descended five flights of stairs to the main deck. The 'Moliqpaq' was a mobile caisson and was floated into position and then sunk on an artificially dredged and submerged island. This enabled drilling to take place year round. The caisson stood on a base 364 feet square and rose ninety-five feet above that. Given the mobility, it could be used in up to seventy feet of water.

Accommodating one hundred residents, with dining for fourty-eight at one sitting, this Arctic behemoth took a long time to explore. We climbed down to the sand base underneath. There seemed to be room down there for a couple of football games to take place. We were now standing under the Arctic Ocean on an artificial island; the addition of some artificial sun and some chairs and umbrellas would have completed the weird effect! The drill could penetrate to a depth of 20,000 feet.

Remaining there until 4 p.m., we then flew back to 'Tuk' in the Bell 212. Ice ridges climbed to as high as 30-40 feet and we passed more open water. Near one open lead, a mother polar bear and her cub were playing, but they were frightened by the noisy 212. The ceiling remained at 500' all the way, with clouds and fog below that. The chopper was in and out of it, trying to remain VFR. Pat said they rarely had better ceilings. My ploy to get Bob to accompany me on this trip was thc promise of the midnight sun. We had not seen it once yet!

Back at the Nalluk base we ate the usual boring meal—smoked salmon followed by veal schnitzel with pan-fries; prosciuto for the veal. Fruit followed for dessert, accompanied by a lemon-meringue pie and ice cream. The next day we had to go into town, just to feel that there was still a normal Arctic life here!

Father LeMer, at 'Tuk', was known to me from my friendship with Fr. Metayer in Cambridge Bay. He had been one of the old school of Oblates and remembered me as the one who had helped Fr. Metayer in his last year. We had an involved talk on the changing Arctic, especially with reference to land claims. Most people who have spent any time in the Arctic have strong opinions, and these older Oblates were well known for their individuality and strength of character. Fr. LeMer was no exception and was outspoken, holding controversial views on modern development.

Fr. LeMer shared an idea which had never occurred to me. He felt that the Oblates who came to the Arctic after World War II had all had enough of authority, even in their own church. Many had lived through the Nazi occupation of Belgium and were rebels. In earlier days, he agreed with me, there had been some primitive 'soul-catching', but later there was a more genuine interest in the language and culture. Many of these Oblates were happy to live in the Arctic, away even from the authority of their own church.

The room in Father LeMer's small house was now filled with cigarette smoke. Bob was fast asleep in his chair but he soon woke up and offered an important observation:

"The Nalluk will soon be serving supper."

Of course we could not afford to miss a meal. As I thanked Fr. LeMer I said good-bye to someone who personified an Arctic era for me. I retained tremendous respect for some of these pioneers, who travelled vast distances, learned new languages and were much loved, in a genuine fashion, by the Inuit.

On May 11th, we attempted to fly to Herschel Island ourselves. We had been up in the weather office at Tuktoyaktuk; it was not encouraging:

Nicholson—partially obscured, 400' ceiling, visibility 5 miles in fog.

Cape Young—200' obscured, 1/8 mile visibility in fog.

Clinton Point—broken layer at 300', 2 miles in fog.

Cape Parry—obscured at 300', blowing snow, fog, 3/4 mile visibility.

All the temperatures and dewpoints were within one degree of each other—something no pilot likes to hear. The winds were up to 25 knots in most places. Out to the west it looked a little better and at the 'Munaksee' the ceiling was at 1000', the wind was 7 knots and the dewpoint and temperature spread 3°. There were low points at Shingle Point and at the Esso Oil rig. At Shingle Point, temperature and dewpoint were identical. I elected to go to Herschel, and try passing that area slightly to the north. The helicopter pilots thought it might be O.K. There was an ice strip out at Herschel where we hoped to land.

After take-off we headed off at 215 degrees on the directional gyro. The magnetic compass works somewhat in this part of the Arctic. I had to add 10 degrees for the northerly wind. Blowing at 25-30 knots from 350 degrees, it needed to be calculated in for our navigation. I was able to track outbound on the 'Tuk' ADF and the Esso VOR. Outbound cross-wind tracking is a good test of nerves! Just south of Garry Island we hit some really low stuff and the temperature and dewpoint met; right on my windscreen! Everything iced up and I lost VOR, ADF, and VHF radio. Time to head home!

I did a 180° turn on instruments at 300' above the sea

ice and back-tracked on a reciprocal heading. I calculated that I would need another 10° of northerly heading because I would be into the headwind longer. I was able to get Kenting Oil rig on the radio, in passing, just to let them know what I was planning. What I really wanted to say was: "HELP!" However, there was little anyone else could do for us. By lowering to 200' I was able to clear the windshield of ice, but there were still no communications to Tuktoyaktuk. We were probably too low.

Crossing the mid-point of Richards Island, we tried to map read. It was almost impossible. The land, sea ice and sky merged in one white haze. In the worst eventuality, we could have landed on the sea ice below but we would not have been able to tie the plane down in a 30 knot wind—to cut through six feet of sea ice would not have been possible for us. To make a survival camp there did not look feasible; there was not enough snow to make an igloo and wait out the weather.

Just as I was beginning to get seriously concerned, we passed over some aerials, clearing them by 100'. I remembered them from the way out. We had crossed over land by now, but it was hard to tell from the plane. This meant we were right on track, through some miracle, and not far from Tuktoyaktuk. When we were close by Esso's VOR, I was able to pick it up again. Six miles from 'Tuk' the ADF came 'alive' and we were able to find the airport in blowing snow. It can be very hard to see an airport at all in those conditions. The airport operator greeted us with:

"Wind is at 25 knots gusting to 35 from 90° to the runway. Landing at your discretion."

I was so tired I could only figure that she meant I could land wherever I wanted to. I landed on the runway, once again exceeding the Maule's stated crosswind maximum. I was too exhausted to go around and approach for a landing on the taxiway. As I landed I began to appreciate how close we had been to not making it back at all.

On the ground, Carter Kelly watched with amusement. His only comment was:

"Well I'm just heading in for some supper; want to come?"

The plane was tied down in no time and we gratefully went in for a shower, and another excellent meal. I felt that I had aged ten years in this one flight. My logbook just says "1.2 hours flying", and "'Tuk' to Shingle Point and return." Bob did not seem worried however, and muttered something about it being a different world up there. We drove in with Carter and ate smoked salmon, stuffed eggs and lemon meringue pie.

When supper was over, I tried to analyze my mistakes and cornered Pat Casey. His only comment was that helicopter flying was so different that it was hard for him to set my limits. He had no idea how angry I was with myself for attempting a flight in such marginal weather. He flew in it all the time with the helicopter.

We nearly overstayed our welcome at Nalluk Base! We had not intended to stay so long but the weather socked in and forced us to abandon our plan to fly over to Holman Island. I had already paid for a barrel of avgas over there, but now we had to go south again. The avgas was never collected. Checking the weather in the morning gave us the following report:

YUB SA 1900 -X E35 OVC 11/2S-035/-8/-10/32/13/963/S7SC3 DRFTING SNW

What this meant to a pilot was that it was not a good day for flying! Looking out of the window it was obvious; nothing but blowing snow. The blizzard stayed all day and one Twin Otter did make it in, but the ground crew had to crack ice off the plane before the return flight to Inuvik.

Finally, the following morning, it was -12° Centigrade in Tuktoyaktuk and there was a ceiling of 1500'. Inuvik and the Mackenzie route south were open. Carter Kelly borrowed a Herman Nelson heater, to pre-warm the aircraft engine, and soon we were on our way. Right after take-off I began to wonder who measured the ceiling. At 700' we were in ice fog and picking up rime ice. I stayed below it and by talking to a Twin Otter pilot found out that it would lift soon. Inuvik was only 80 miles away anyway. I held an outbound VOR and ADF heading for ten minutes at 500', occasionally losing ground contact altogether. Soon it cleared though, and we saw sunshine for the first time in a week. With some landing breaks for gas, it took 10 hours to fly back to the 108 Mile airstrip, in central British Columbia. We arrived home thc next evening.

It was May 15th, and all this had taken 12 days. It seemed as if we had been away for weeks!

Epilogue

After a twelve year association with the Arctic I still had the 'polar passion'. Flying and practicing medicine in the north had enabled me to live and travel in an area of Canada which is out of reach to most people. Getting to know the original inhabitants of this country was a privilege, and in experiencing first hand the 'magic' of the far north, I felt that I had been very fortunate. Like many other 'ex-northerners', I still spend time planning ways to get back up there, see old friends and revisit some of the most intriguing places on this planet.

Snowshoes & Stethoscopes

ORDER FORM

To order "Snowshoes & Stethoscopes" mail this form to:

Daedalus Publishing
Box 489, Nelson
British Columbia, Canada,
V1L 5R3

Name ______________________________

Address ____________________________

City ______________ Prov./State __________

Country ____________ Postal Code __________

Please send me _______ copies (y) of Snowshoes & Stethoscopes at $16.95 (Cdn) $_____

Shipping and handling: _____
include $3.50 for the first book,
$1 for each additional book.

Add 7% GST _____

Total amount enclosed $_____
Cheque or money order only.